PROMOTING MEN'S HEALTH —

AN ESSENTIAL BOOK FOR NURSES

Other titles published by Ausmed Publications

Nursing the Person with Cancer
Edited by Gordon Poulton

Nursing Documentation: writing what we do
Edited by Jennifer Richmond

Spirituality: The Heart of Nursing
Edited by Professor Susan Ronaldson

Rethinking Dementia — an Australian approach
Edited by Sally Garratt and Elery Hamilton-Smith

Thinking Management: Focusing on People
Edited by Jean Anderson

Caring for People with Problem Behaviours
Bernadette Keane and Carolyn Dixon

Asian Mothers, Australian Birth
Edited by Pranee Liamputtong Rice

Unique and Ordinary: Reflections on Living and Dying in a Nursing Home
Rosalie Hudson and Jennifer Richmond

Geriatric Medicine
Len Gray, Michael Woodward, Ron Scholes and David Fonda

Urinary Incontinence
David Fonda and Cynthea Wellings

PROMOTING MEN'S HEALTH —

AN ESSENTIAL BOOK FOR NURSES

Edited by Tom Laws

Foreword by Professor Alan Pearson

AUSMED PUBLICATIONS

MELBOURNE

Australasian Health Education Systems Pty Ltd
(ACN 005 611 626)
trading as
Ausmed Publications
275–277Mount Alexander Road
Ascot Vale, Victoria 3032, Australia

First published July 1998

Further copies of this book and of all other Ausmed publications are available from the Distribution Manager, Ausmed Publications, PO Box 4086, Melbourne University, Victoria 3052, Australia.
Telephone +61 3 9375 7311.
Fax +61 3 9375 7299.
E-mail ausmed@ausmed.com.au
Home page www.ausmed.com.au

National Library of Australia Cataloguing-in-Publication data:
Promoting men's health: an essential book for nurses
Includes index.
ISBN 0 9587171 1 7.

1. Men - Health and hygiene - Australia. 2. Men - Diseases - Australia. 3. Fathers - Health and hygiene - Australia. 4. Health promotion - Australia.
I. Laws, Tom, 1955-.

613.042340994

Edited by Robyn Whiteley and John Collins, The WC Company Pty Ltd
Cover, design and typesetting by Colorperception Pty Ltd

Text set in 10pt Garamond
Printed in Australia by Hyde Park Press

FOREWORD

Alan Pearson

The rapid development of women-centred health services in most Western countries in the past decade arose out of many years of lobbying and consciousness raising by women's groups. The same can be said about changes in approaches to the schooling of girls. The result is a range of health services designed specially for women and a success rate in secondary schooling for girls which far exceeds that of boys. As we approach the end of the twentieth century, we can take some pride in the gains made in meeting the needs of women and in removing, at least in part, the dominance of male leaders and male-oriented service provision.

But what of men, of that half of the population who have, according to the dominant discourses in gender politics, been the recipients of educational and health services that have been designed predominantly to meet *their* needs? The response to such a question is indeed intriguing. Men have a shorter life span than women; men have higher morbidity rates than women; men use health services less often than women (even those services which are not especially women oriented); men take more risks with their health than women; men are much less receptive of positive health messages and thus less likely to change their lifestyle than women; males do less well than females at school and in higher education; young males are much more likely to commit suicide than females — the list goes on.

In the preface to *Men's Health: The Forgotten Issue*, published by Ausmed Publications in 1993, I argued that:

> Men are reluctant to use mainstream health services because, just like women, they find them cold, clinical, threatening and dehumanising. While many argue that health services and systems have been established by men to serve men, it is time to challenge this. Men's health has indeed become a forgotten issue. The bookshelves are stacked with work on women's health, but the literature on men and their health is still tiny.

Although little has changed in the design and lack of person-centred approaches in health service delivery, I am pleased to see that the literature on men's health has begun to develop apace. This book is a fine example of the growth in the literature and I am delighted to have been asked to write the foreword. The authors of the book are representative of the growing number of outstanding researchers, practitioners and social commentators who have taken men's plight seriously in terms of their health and moved on to creatively develop deeper understandings of what it means to be a man and what role health plays in men's constructions of their lives.

While the focus of the book is on promoting health amongst men, the contents are not overly focused on classical approaches to health education. What it is to be a man in Australia is sensitively and incisively explored in Section One.

In Section Two, titled 'Men's health on the move', approaches to developing health in men through designing and offering men's health programs, raising a consciousness of men's needs in nurses and other health professionals and supporting healthy lifestyles for older men are examined. The role of men in family life is addressed in Section Three and Section Four focuses on current issues in the field of men's health.

This book brings together a strong group of scholars and practitioners with a broad range of interests and expertise. I congratulate them on the clarity of this work, for making such a significantly original contribution to the literature on men and, most of all, for their continuing efforts to ensure that men's health ceases to be a marginalised, forgotten issue.

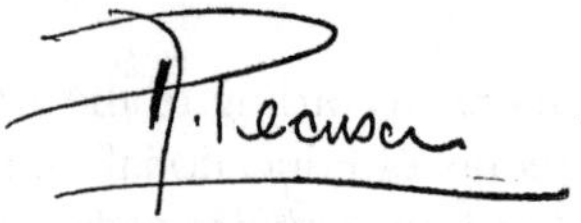

Alan Pearson, RN, ONC, DipNEd, DANS, MSc, PhD, FCN (NSW), FINE, FRCNA, FRCN, is Professor of Clinical Nursing at The University of Adelaide and Director of the Joanna Briggs Institute for Evidence-based Nursing and Midwifery at the Royal Adelaide Hospital, both of which are in Adelaide, South Australia.

Adelaide
March 1998

CONTENTS

THIS BOOK IS DEDICATED TO
JULIE, DAVID AND HENRY.

INTRODUCTION

Tom Laws

Literature focusing on men's health is a relatively new social phenomenon. As such it is worth outlining some of the arguments that have supported the move for social change in this area. The recent emergence of a men's health movement and the development of public health policy have not been created out of a need to match the resources devoted toward improving the health status of women. Rather, the movement has been built upon the premise that men have particular health needs and problems. These problems stem not only from the biological differences that exist between the sexes but from the way in which men are socialised and exhibit masculine traits. For example, men accept higher levels of risk to their health than women and are less likely to acknowledge that they have a health problem.

The inability of our health system to react to these problems has been seen as cause for concern only recently. There has been a general assumption that because a health care system is not seen to be meeting women's needs it must somehow be meeting the needs of men. The fact is that men die younger than women, access health facilities less often than women and have a poorer level of understanding of health promotion and the treatment of illness.

These problems have been attributed, to some extent, to the way in which the health care system has been dominated by the biomedical model. This model focuses on treating the disease rather than focusing on the individual or groups within society. The cost of this medical treatment has been rising for many years and is a major concern for any government. The restoration of health, once illness has occurred, is a more costly approach to illness management than are methods that focus on prevention.

Researchers of public health are now more than ever concerned with identifying the health care needs of groups and individuals within communities so as to plan for more efficient and effective means of promoting health and wellbeing. The emphasis of this approach is illness prevention and management of health problems within the community not in institutions.

It is against this background that this book was conceived. The purpose of the text is to inform health professionals and those interested in men's health of the current issues, research findings and strategies used by health workers to improve men's health.

The book is structured into four themes. The first explores the ways in which men and their masculine traits shape their health status. The second looks at strategies that have been effective in promoting men's health and their sense of wellbeing. The third considers the extent to which men are able and willing to be involved in addressing important health care issues within the family.

The chapters within these three themes have been written by researchers of men's health and health professionals working with men in the community. The final theme centres on the personal reflections of three men in relation to their experience of a surviving a life-threatening illness. Their assessment of the treatment options they were offered, the ability of health workers to meet their needs and their reactions to illness are compelling reading for anyone with an interest in health care.

This book represents a unique approach to men's health. It provides contemporary information and analysis from experts, who are intimately involved in promoting health care, as well as a rich account of men's lived experiences.

Section One

THE AUSTRALIAN MALE IN FOCUS

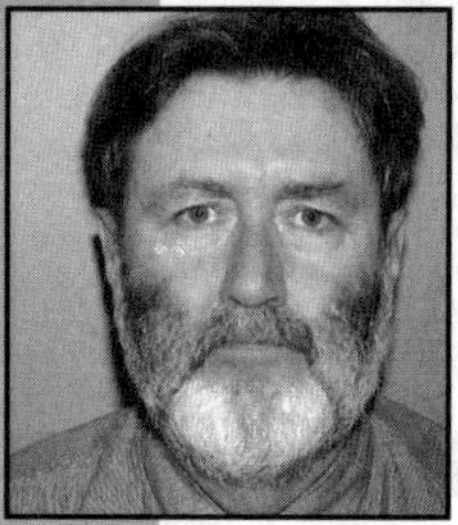

ALLAN K. HUGGINS

Master of Education, Advanced Diploma of Adolescent Development, Certificate of Technology, Member of the British Association for Behavioural Psychotherapy

Senior Lecturer and Director, Men's Health Teaching and Research Unit, School of Public Health, Curtin University, Perth, Western Australia

The Men's Health Teaching and Research Unit is the first of its kind in any university in Australia. It offers a certificate course in men's health taught both internally and externally around Australia and in New Zealand. This course has recently been accredited by the Royal Australian College of General Practitioners. The Unit is also involved in a range of men's health issues around Australia. In 1995 Allan Huggins was appointed to the Men's Health National Policy Development Committee which drafted the first National Men's Health Policy Document. His teaching and research interests include men's health epidemiology, policy development, tertiary education development and risk behaviour, including self-harm and suicide; the social determinants of health; and health services law and ethics. Of this chapter Allan said, *'I thought that writing this chapter might provide a contribution to both informing and directing current and future endeavours in the area of men's health in Australia.'*

Chapter 1

The Australian male: illness, injury and death by socialisation — a paradox of health inequalities

INTRODUCTION

Many men's health problems in Australia are preventable. They are broad public health issues such as lifestyle, health-risk behaviour and poor health care service utilisation. Although there have been a few gains in men's health in the last 20 years, especially in the cardiovascular and smoking arenas, men's health is still not being taken seriously enough by medical professionals, health administrators and health planners. For example there is almost a complete lack of men's health studies taught in Schools of Nursing throughout Australian universities.

Improving men's health in Australia depends on a number of prerequisites. These include the recognition that:

- men's poor health status and health risk are an outcome of risk behaviour;
- men's poor health outcomes should not taken for granted as a cultural norm;
- men's health problems are not going to be solved by biomedicine alone;
- men's health and behaviour is not predominantly predetermined by biogenetic factors — lifestyle and socialisation are some of the most important factors;
- men's health is very much influenced by construct issues such as male socialisation and the models of masculinity that predominate in the Australian culture;

- the unreasonable expectations placed on young men to conform to male stereotypic behaviour result in health-risk behaviour which is detrimental to health; and
- ultimately, men are the only people who can improve men's health by being given permission to participate in problem solving and the decision-making process

The traditional models of masculinity and identity, with their associated patterns of behaviour, which are dominant within the Australian and New Zealand cultures, are detrimental and injurious to boys and men. There is some evidence to suggest that males who adopt a traditional masculine role are less receptive to health promotion messages and are more inclined to adopt health risk behaviour, (Smith, 1994). If men's health is to improve, traditional models of masculinity need to be seriously challenged.

MEN'S HEALTH STATUS

Although some issues in men's health have received attention, and some gains have been made, for example, premature mortality from heart disease has been partially reduced, and male deaths from lung cancer are beginning to decline, there are still major concerns about men's health status which are not being tackled systematically in the Australian and New Zealand communities. Among many other issues, male youth suicide in New Zealand is not being systematically approached by health authorities. In Australia there is still no political will to address development of a men's health policy even in the face of mounting epidemiological evidence (Huggins, 1995; Mathers, 1994; ABS National Health Survey, 1989–90).

Perhaps more substantial evidence has been presented by Templer et al. (1993), who examined male-to-female life expectancy ratios in 161 countries and found evidence that alcohol misuse accounted for an appreciable amount of the male life years lost. Similarly, based on information collated from 12 large studies in the USA, Waldron (1988) posits that, for adults, approximately half of the sex differences in total mortality could be attributed to smoking, with higher propositions at younger ages and lower propositions at older ages. Up to 50 per cent of mortality from the ten leading causes of death in the USA may be related to behaviour such as:

- smoking,
- use of alcohol and drugs,
- poor diet,
- reckless driving,
- maladaptive responses to stress and
- non-compliance with medication.

Primarily this is men's behaviour in a nutshell and is not a function of their biology but a function of their socialisation (Hamburg et al., 1985, cited in Strodl, 1994).

GENDER ISSUES

Certainly men's health and wellbeing have been gaining more attention in the community. Gender issues have become more important because it is now recognised that men and women within the same Australian culture have very different experiences of personal health status. Health-risk behaviour is greatly influenced by the 'genderising' process, especially for young men and boys. Health outcomes are greatly influenced by what gender behaviours happen to be adopted, or imposed, within a given culture.

Men not only die younger than women, but also suffer higher rates of injury and most illnesses. Men participate, to a much greater extent, in health-risk behaviours, access health services differently (and to a much lesser extent than women), and are generally not receptive to health promotion messages. Men's health (like women's health) is increasingly being recognised as an issue that is socially constructed and depends greatly on how men and their community define masculinity. The feminist movement in the last 30 years goes part of the way to explaining why women are now more in control of their own health and personal identity. In Australia and New Zealand national sex differential epidemiological evidence is now available to support this (Mathers, 1994, [Australia]; Raeburn, 1995 [New Zealand]).

A surge of recent research is questioning the often-held view that gender differentials in mortality and morbidity rates are primarily biological (Manuk and Polefrone, 1987; Ramey and Ramwell, 1984; Stacey and Olesen, 1993; Rodin and Ickovics, 1990; Waldron, 1988; Hugo, 1986; Strickland, 1988). While not denying the importance of biological differences in patterns of mortality and morbidity, an increasing body of evidence points to the importance of behavioural and environmental factors. Harrison et al. (1989), after examining gender differences in mortality rates throughout life, concluded that, after childhood, biological factors alone cannot account for the increased longevity of women.

The most striking example of this mortality excess for men over women includes:

- ischaemic heart disease overall 253 per cent higher
- suicide overall 252 per cent higher
- lung cancer overall 223 per cent higher
- motor vehicle accidents overall 171 per cent higher (see Tables 1.3 and 1.4)

Australian men's life expectancy in 1990 was 6.1 years less than women's and this differential has doubled since the turn of the century.

Table 1.1 Average life expectancy for males and females in Australia

Year	Female	Male	Difference
1901	58.2	55.2	3.0
1990	80.0	73.9	6.1
INCREASE	21.8	18.7	

(Source: Social Indicators Number 5, 1992, ABS)

Interestingly the New Zealand profile is very similar.

Young males from lower socioeconomic circumstances have excess mortality and an array of factors leading them to participate in risk-taking behaviours which are reflected significantly in state and national injury and suicide statistics. Throughout their lives men are more likely than women to die from a whole range of causes. For example, young men aged 15–24 are more than three times as likely to die in motor vehicle accidents as young women and more than six times as likely to die of suicide. Men aged 25–64 have a death rate nearly twice that of women in the same age range, with major contributors being heart disease and suicide (both three and a half times higher), lung cancer (over three times as high), and motor vehicle accidents (almost three times as high) (Mathers, 1994). Men aged 65 years and above have a death rate more than one and a half times greater than their female contemporaries. These men have higher death rates than women from all major causes of death, including genitourinary disease. For example, older men die from lung cancer at nearly five times the rate of women, of suicide at nearly four times the rate, and of bronchitis/emphysemalasthma at nearly three times the rate.
The following tables (Tables 1.2 to 1.5) provide a graphic illustration of these points.

Table 1.2 Cause of death for the 0–14-year age group

Cause of death	% difference
Accidental drowning	males 171% higher than females
Sudden infant death syndrome	males 59% higher than females
Motor vehicle traffic accidents	males 53% higher than females
Circulatory system anomalies	males 32% higher than females
Chromosomal anomalies	males 44% higher than females

(Source: The Australian Institute of Health and Welfare, 1992)

Table 1.3 Cause of death for the 15–24-year age group

Cause of death	% difference
Suicide	males 325% higher than females
Motor vehicle traffic accidents	males 214% higher than females
Other injuries	males 266 % higher than females
Drug dependence	males 83% higher than females
Cancers	males 60% higher than females

(Source: The Australian Institute of Health and Welfare, 1992)

Table 1.4 Cause of death for the 25–64 year age group

Cause of death	% difference
Ischaemic heart disease	males 253% higher than females
Suicide	males 252% higher than females
Lung cancer	males 223% higher than females
Motor vehicle/traffic accident	males 170% higher than females
Stomach cancer	males 130% higher than females
Stroke	males 34% higher than females

(Source: The Australian Institute of Health and Welfare, 1992)

Table 1.5 Cause of death for the 65 years and over age group

Cause of death	% difference
Lung cancer	males 389% higher than females
Bronchitis/emphysema/asthma	males 197% higher than females
Stomach cancer	males 137% higher than females
Ischaemic heart disease	males 70% higher than females
Injury and poisoning	males 64% higher than females
Other cancers	males 57% higher than females
Diabetes	males 25% higher than females
Stroke	males 6% higher than females

(Source: The Australian Institute of Health and Welfare, 1992)

Women use health services at a higher rate than men, except for injuries. Hospitalisation, general practitioner utilisation, and other health provider utilisation, for most of men's lives, is 40 per cent lower than for women, even when obstetric admissions are allowed for (National Health Strategy Research Paper No1, DHHCS, Canberra 1992). Men have significantly higher rates of cardiovascular disease: they are 54 per cent more likely to suffer from hypertension, 48 per cent more likely to be overweight, 32 per cent more likely to smoke, 15 per cent more likely to have a high plasma cholesterol; and 106 per cent more likely to consume excess alcohol.

It is only when men become much older that their hospitalisation rates increase dramatically. Men do not like to admit they are sick or injured for it flies in the face of their socialisation, which dictates that they should be strong, emotionally flat, non-expressive of pain and feelings, and should certainly never cry or get distressed. Men are encouraged, at the extreme end of this process, to deny pain, remain stoic, cope with suffering and develop an unemotional language of response. Many doctors do not recognise that men need more time in a consultation to unravel some of their medical and personal issues

Men are the victims here, a bi-product of what someone once called the hard masculine culture of Australia: 'If you don't measure up, you are not a real man or you're not quite a man'. In order to cope with these high expectations many men resort to the use of social drugs. Excessive alcohol consumption is associated strongly with definitions of masculinity in Australia and New Zealand.

Men and women are socialised differently in almost all cultures, and both have been losers in that process. Aspects of men's socialisation have had a major impact on health-risk behaviour, mental health and their sense of wellbeing. Excessive competition, unrealistic and unattainable models of masculinity, poor self-esteem, lack of meaningfulness, poor identity formation and a lack of sustainable role models, are some of the culprits that have left many men in their teens, early twenties, after the age of 45 and after retirement feeling they have reached their use-by date.

Tragically many younger men are feeling they have reached their 'use-by date' and are 'taking themselves off the shelves'. If you think that all of this is a little far-fetched, remember that Australia and New Zealand have some of the highest suicide rates in the world and that in Australia more young men die of suicide than road accidents and in New Zealand the greatest killers of young men are road accidents and suicide.

For Aboriginal and Torres Strait Islander men, the picture is grim and depressing. An Aboriginal male born in 1992 was approximately three times as likely to die before the age of five as a non-indigenous male child. The Aboriginal child's life expectancy would also be around 55 years — between 16 and 18 years shorter than for his non-Aboriginal contemporaries. Successive governments have failed to solve this issue and our poor record in relation to indigenous health has now reached the notice of the international community.

Changing the gender role definition of the traditional Australian male has positive implications for health, yet it seems to many in authority, both politically and in the health bureaucracy, to be 'pie in the sky' .The definition of what it means to be a man in Australia has to change before things can improve. If men adopted some traits that have been traditionally associated with women our society would be healthier and more cohesive. Many men find this argument too disturbing to contemplate, mainly, I think, because of their blinkered commitment to mainstream masculinity and their unconscious need to defend it.

There is a dangerous assumption in the Australian health community that male health-related needs are already being met. A few years ago this was classically illustrated by a court testimony of Dr Stephen Duckett, the then Director of Policy and Planning for the Victorian Health Department, when he stated:

> . . . one would hope that existing services are meeting someone's needs and if they're not meeting women's needs they are presumably meeting men's needs.

This notion, that just because services are available they are automatically and magically meeting needs, is a fallacy. The planning of health services very rarely takes into account gender issues, especially as they relate to boys and men. Health policy makers automatically think in terms of women's health or Aboriginal health or children's health but they do not think of, or indeed consider, men's health.

RAISING AWARENESS

The National Men's Health Conference held in Melbourne in 1995 was the first step in developing a shared better understanding of the social, behavioural and environmental factors that are affecting men's health. Over 500 delegates attended the conference, representing such fields as medicine, nursing, sociology, community health and consumer groups. Specific population groups, such as Aboriginal and Torres Strait Islander men, men from non-English-speaking backgrounds and gay men, were also well represented.

The issues covered at the conference were varied, ranging across physical health, mental health, socialisation, sexuality and the impacts of differing cultural and socioeconomic backgrounds. This conference provided an initial point of consultation with the community on the development of a national men's health policy, allowing delegates to comment on areas of priority for men's health. This was an important part of the proceedings. The key areas identified at the conference, included:

- the negative impacts of male socialisation on risk-taking behaviour and in creating an unwillingness for men to talk about health or seek help;
- the need for broad education strategies on the full range of men's health issues, involving schools, the media and workplaces; and
- the need to better target existing services to improve outcomes for men.

CONCLUSION

The overwhelming impression that one gets after looking seriously at men's health in Australia and New Zealand is that, first, a great deal more research needs to be done in the area of men's health and, secondly, that men's health is in crisis and is not going to improve unless some fundamental issues are confronted in the Australian and New Zealand cultures. The very definition of traditional masculinity and the way boys and young men are socialised in our Australian and New Zealand multicultural societies is having an adverse impact on health status and participation in health-risk behaviour. The health indicators are there for all to see. The important fact to remember is that most of these health issues relating to men are potentially avoidable. They are not just a function of testosterone and the well-worn excuse that men behave the way they do because that is how it is pre-ordained.

Masculinity needs reworking, restructuring and redefining. However this job needs to be done by men in consultation with other men (and women). This process has already started in Australia with the emergence of university courses in men's health and men's studies and the reworking of some gender equity policies statements, at a state level, especially in education

This is the challenge, as yet unmet, for men's health promotion. Biomedicine has a part to play in this process but it is not the solution. A national men's health policy is also an imperative in the same way as a women's health policy was and still is an imperative.

References

Australian Bureau of Statistics (ABS): *National Health Survey 1989–90.* Canberra: AGPS.

Australian Institute of Health and Welfare (1992): *Australian Health 1992.* Canberra: AGPS.

Hamburg D, Elliot G and Parron D (eds) (1982): *Health and Behaviour: Frontiers in Research in the Behavioural Sciences.* Washington, DC: National Academy Press.

Harrison J, Chin J and Ficarrotto T (1989): Warning: Masculinity May Be Dangerous to Your Health: In: Kimmel MS and Messner MA (eds): *Men's Lives.* New York: Macmillan.

Huggins AK (1995): Men's health as a serious issue not being taken seriously enough: The need for a cultural change in the way we view masculinity and health. Unpublished paper, presented at the Men's Health Conference, Melbourne, 1995.

Hugo G (1986): *Australia's Changing Population.* Melbourne: Oxford University Press.

Mathers C (1994): *Health Differentials among Adult Australians Aged 25–64 Years.* Australian Institute of Health and Welfare.

Raeburn J (1995): Review of Men's Health: New Zealand. Auckland: Department of Psychiatry and Behavioural Studies, Auckland University.

Ramey ER and Ramwell P (1984): The Relationship of the Sex Hormone/Prostagladin Interaction to Female and Male Longevity. In Gold EB (ed.): *The Changing Risk of Disease in Women: An Epidemiologic Approach*. pp. 25–36.

Rodin J and Ickovics JR (1990): Women's health: Review and research agenda as we approach the 21st century. *American Psychologist* 45: 1018–1034.

Smith J (1994): *Men's Health Project Report.* Pilbara Public Health Unit.

Stacey M and Oleson V (1993): Introduction. *Social Science and Medicine* 36: 1–5.

Strickland BR (1988): Sex-related differences in health and illness. *Psychology of Women Quarterly* 12: 381–399.

Strodl E (1994): *A Review of Men's Health Literature: Biological vs Behaviour Factors.* Darling Downs Health Authority: Queensland Health.

Templer DI, Griffin PR and Hintze J (1993): Gender life expectancy and alcohol: An international perspective. *The International Journal of the Addictions* 28: 1613–1620.

Waldron I (1988): Gender and Health-related Behaviour. In: Gochman David S (ed.): *Health Behaviour: Emerging Research Perspectives.* New York: Plenum Press.

Suggested reading

Archer M (1989): *Culture and Agency: The Place of Culture in Social Theory.* Cambridge: Cambridge University Press.

Binns CW, Knowles SS and Blaze-Temple D (1987): Is education enough? The drinking and driving practices of 17–30 year old males. *Australian Drug and Alcohol Review* 6: 253–264.

Brand RR (1993): Men at risk. *Australian Family Physician* 22:1343–1348.

Buchbinder (1995): *Masculinities and Identities.* Melbourne: Melbourne University Press.

Eisler RM and Blalock JA (1991): Masculine gender role stress: Implications for the assessment of men. *Clinical Psychology Review* 2: 45–60.

Foreman MD (1986): Cardiovascular disease: A men's health hazard. *Nursing Clinics of North America* 21: 65–73.

Hafner J (1986). Stereotyping of men: Effects on mental health. *Dulwich Centre Review*, pp. 78–84.

Hiscock-Corney LS (1989): Health and safety issues for Victorian farm workers. *The Australian Journal of Advanced Nursing* 6: 25–28.

Levant RF (1990): Psychological services designed for men: A psychoeducational approach. *Psychotherapy* 27: 309–315.

Levy S and Pierce JP (1990): Predictors of marijuana use and uptake among teenagers in Sydney, Australia. *The International Journal of the Addictions* 25: 1179–1193.

Manuck SB and Polefrone JM (1987): Psychophysiologic Reactivity in Women. In: Eaker ED, Packard B, Wenger NK, Clarkson TB and Tyroler HA (eds): *Coronary Heart Disease in Women*. New York: Haymarket Doyma, pp. 164–171.

National Health and Medical Research Council (1994): *Men and Mental Health*.

National Heart Foundation (1989): *Risk Factor Prevalence Survey*

Ossler CC (1986): Men's work environments and health risks. *Nursing Clinics of North America* 21: 25–36.

Renwick MY (1986): Occupational hazards in agriculture in northern New South Wales: Farmers' perceptions and experiences. *Journal of Occupational Health and Safety — Australia and New Zealand* 2: 497–506.

Ryan GA, Barker JM, Wright JN and McLean AJ (1992): Human factors in rural road crashes. *Australian Journal of Public Health* 16: 269–276.

Swensen G, Serafino S and Thomson N (1995): *Suicide in Western Australia, 1983–1992.* Perth: Health Department of Western Australia.

Verbrugge LM and Steiner RP (1985): Prescribing drugs to men and women. *Health Psychology* 4: 79–98.

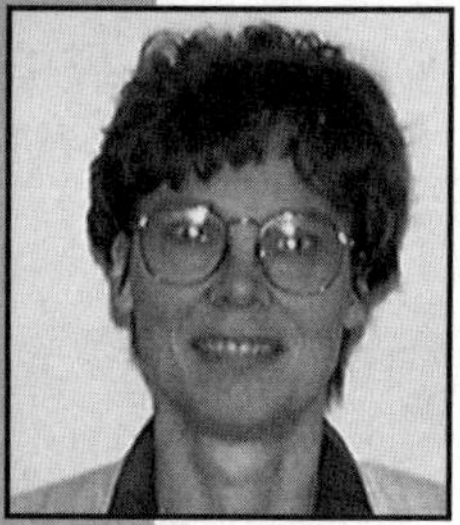

CHRISTINE TAYLOR

Registered Nurse, Bachelor of Applied Science (Advanced Nursing), Master of Health Science Education, Member of the College of Nursing (New South Wales)
Lecturer, Department of Nursing Practice, Australian Catholic University, Sydney

Christine has had a wide variety of clinical nursing experience both in Australia and overseas. At present she is a doctoral candidate and her research activities include, in collaboration with Ailsa Stewart, an investigation into the health behaviour and attitudes of Australian males. Christine is a member of the College of Nursing (NSW), and of the Australasian and New Zealand Association for Medical Education. She is also a reviewer for the *Australian Journal of Advanced Nursing*.

AILSA STEWART

Registered Nurse, Acute Respiratory Certificate, Diploma of Teaching (Nursing), Master of Arts, Fellow of the College of Nursing (New South Wales), Fellow of the Royal College of Nursing, Australia
Senior Lecturer, Department of Nursing Practice, Australian Catholic University, Sydney

Ailsa has a wide clinical experience and has published previously in the area of culture care nursing. She has conducted research into health promotion and primary health care and is at present, with Christine Taylor, researching Australian men's health behaviours and attitudes. Ailsa is a Fellow of both the Royal Australian College of Nursing and the NSW College of Nursing. She is also a member of the Australian Health Promotion Professionals Association.

ROBERT J. PARKER

Diploma of Education; Bachelor of Education; Master of Education; Fellow of the Australian College of Health, Physical Education and Recreation
Senior Lecturer in Human Movement Science, Department of Human Movement, Australian Catholic University, Sydney

Robbie is the author of four books and has contributed to several publications used in secondary schools. He has presented at many conferences in Australia and overseas. He is at present completing his doctorate on the efficacy of exercise on fat loss. He is also investigating the health and fitness levels of school-aged children in NSW, and has just completed seven major reports on the results of the NSW Youth Sports Injury Survey 1994–95. In 1995 Robbie was appointed as a clinical consultant in Sports Medicine to the New Children's Hospital Institute of Sports Medicine, Westmead, Sydney. He is the chairperson of the NSW Fitness Advisory Council and a member of the Australian Fitness Accreditation Council. Robbie has also represented Australia in Rugby.

Chapter 2

'MACHISMO' AS A BARRIER TO HEALTH PROMOTION IN AUSTRALIAN MALES

There is a significant difference between men and women when it comes to health. Compared with women, men do not live as long and they suffer from more illness and disease. Most of the health conditions that men suffer from, and die from, are preventable. However, compared with women, men do not engage in health-promoting behaviours. There has been significant success in developing health promotion programs for women, yet very few programs for men have been successful. There is a need to promote men's health. In order to develop effective health promotion programs to improve the current state of men's health an understanding of men's health behaviour is needed.

Health belief and health promotion models provide frameworks for predicting reasons why people engage in a variety of health behaviours. Within these frameworks gender and psychosociocultural factors are considered to influence behaviour. There are some factors about belonging to a 'male' culture that contribute towards men's poor health. This chapter will explore Australian masculinity and machismo, and its effects upon men's health and behaviours. Machismo will also be discussed as a barrier to health promotion in men. Recommended strategies will be given to assist health professionals to develop effective men's health promotion programs.

Generalisations of male behaviours will be made throughout this chapter. These generalisations are necessary in order to highlight trends and issues in men's health and health behaviours. Patterns that are emerging within the field of men's health can also be explored. Health within the majority of Australian males, and from the dominant culture, will be the focus of this chapter.

HORMONES OR ROLES?

The very nature of being male greatly influences male health behaviours. Accidents, illness and disease become men's health issues when the type of illness or trauma is seen as a manifestation of masculine identity (Allen and Whately, 1986). There are two major types of theories of male behaviour that are relevant to the discussion of male health behaviours:

- biological theories and
- sociocultural theories (Harvey, 1993).

Psychoanalytical theories also seek to explain male behaviour (Connell, 1995; Hargreaves, 1987), however there is scant empirical supporting evidence and the application of such theories is limited in health promotion programs.

Physically men are different from women, both internally and externally. Biological theories state that the physical differences in males create characteristic male behaviour. Testosterone, a sex hormone produced by the testes, decreases the level of 'good' cholesterol in the blood (Smith, 1994). Some studies show that male androgens are arthrogenic, but the studies are inconclusive as the incidence of heart disease varies among countries (Foreman, 1986).

Testosterone also increases aggressiveness and sexual drive in a male (Moir and Jessel, 1991). An Australian naturalist (Smith, 1994) stated that males of most species are more aggressive than females. Much energy is used by the males of most species to reproduce, fight for mates and guard mates, leading to a decreased lifespan. Boles and Tatro (1982:118), in a review of gender studies, stated that

> aggression/violence and success/achievement are central attributes associated with maleness.

Perhaps in the human male this natural aggression, though manifested in other behaviours, is an important factor in the shorter lifespan of males compared with females.

Another biological view, the 'brainsex' theory (Moir and Jessel, 1991), asserts that male and female brains are different, developing differently in utero from about the sixth week, due to the influence of male hormones. Such a difference in brain chemistry and synapse linkage is thought to account for differences in male and female behaviour.

There is strong support for the belief that male behaviour arises out of the unique biological male characteristics. Throughout the world stereotyped male behaviour is extremely similar across a variety of cultures and societies (Bederman, 1995; Leiner, 1994; Radican, 1995; Shapiro, 1992:9). Males are seen as more dominant, more aggressive, more assertive, and engaging in more risk-taking behaviours than females.

Some theorists believe that male behaviour is culturally scripted and socially reinforced, that is, males behave in certain ways due to the influence of society (Foreman, 1986; Harvey, 1993). If socialisation is a major determinant of male behaviour then all cultures and societies must have very similar beliefs about appropriate male behaviour. This raises questions about the common evolution of such scripted behaviour.

In the early evolution of the modern human race men were more physically suited than women to particular tasks — for example, hunting, and protecting mates — because of their greater strength and aggression. Society would have encouraged and reinforced such behaviour in males. Other behaviours desirable to successful hunting would also have been reinforced, such as

- problem solving;
- competitiveness;
- self-reliance;
- planning; and
- physical endurance.

The withholding of emotions such as fear, concern and compassion, would have been beneficial to the coping and survival of the individual male when in situations of extreme duress, such as hunting wild beasts or in battles and conflicts.

There is no doubt that social pressures encourage males to conform to certain behaviours. Socialisation processes reinforce certain innate male behaviours and shape them to the needs of the culture. Gender role theories account for the form in which masculinity is expressed in a society or culture. However, there seems to be an 'essential' maleness that crosses cultural boundaries. Even men who have a nontraditional sex role, such as homosexuals, engage in typically male behaviour such as risk-taking, for example, by engaging in unprotected sex (Leiner, 1994:149).

It is this very nature of 'maleness' that needs to be explored in order to understand male health behaviours. It is extremely unlikely that health workers can change the essential nature of the male but a greater understanding of male behaviour can lead to the development of more effective health programs.

How do the characteristics of male behaviour relate to the poor health statistics for men? There is a need to link the way men die to the way men live (Allen and Whately, 1986:8). To address this issue, the meaning of masculinity in the Australian context needs to explored. In particular, there is a need to focus on the key aspect of 'machismo' within the Australian male culture.

MASCULINITY AND MACHISMO IN THE AUSTRALIAN MALE

Masculinity is defined similarly in a large proportion of cultures, that is, having characteristics of being a man (Macquarie Dictionary, 1991). The word 'macho' is of Spanish origin and means male or masculine. In Australia a common interpretation of 'macho' is 'manly' behaviour. 'Machismo' is often defined as a caricature of 'macho', that is, an attitude of male domination, a display of power (Bilmes, 1992), a masculine display of strength (Macquarie Dictionary, 1985), a need to prove one's virility by daring action (Oxford Dictionary, 1990).

Traditionally, in many cultures, men are dominant, competitive, strong, fit and healthy (Rees et al., 1995). Men are not to cry, show emotions, show fear or ask for help, but are expected to 'soldier' on, be aggressive and take risks (Radican, 1995; Richman, 1982). Brannon (1982) describes the traditional United States of America image of a man as, no 'sissy' stuff, the 'big wheel', the sturdy oak, 'give 'em hell'. Researchers reinforce the stereotyped image of male behaviour by developing tools to measure masculinity. These tools identify behaviours such assertiveness, independence, problem-solving, and emotional inexpressiveness (Bem, 1981;Cunningham and Antwill, 1980; Keisling et al., 1993; Orlofsky et al., 1982; Villemez and Touhey, 1977).

Traditional Australian masculinity differs from other cultures in its focus and emphasis on certain male behaviours. This is due to the unique nature of Australian history. Europeans settled the country as convicts and soldiers and for some time were the country's dominant culture. There were very few women in the settlement. Homosexual acts and bestiality were common (Hughes, 1987). Living conditions and the environment were harsh, and the early settlers nearly starved. To survive as a society men suffered further hardships to explore the surrounding harsh and densely wooded countryside in order to find arable grazing land.

This convict-based, harsh, masculine, pioneering environment led to the development of a specific underlying, or hard, culture. Australian hard culture is described as secular, populist, racist, and masculine (Patience, 1990). This description of Australian hard culture indicates that there is a lack of religious focus in the society, there is a suspicion of intellectuals, a high value is placed on practical knowledge, native Australians are marginalised, and men dominate the public domain (McGrane and Patience, 1993).

In Australia men who publicly show emotion and cry are condemned (Smith, 1994). Think of Bob Hawke when Prime Minister, and cricketer, Kim Hughes. Male social relationships often develop through sport, work and pubs. Socially — for example, at barbecues or in pubs — men will gather in groups to isolate themselves from females, to avoid being considered a 'sissy' by preferring female company or being seen to identify with females. Acceptable male behaviour is where men or boys:

- do not show weakness,
- are homophobic,
- enjoy a beer with their 'mates', and
- in no way wish to exhibit any behaviour considered feminine.

Common expressions in Australia of acceptable male behaviour include 'real men don't eat quiche', and 'Balmain boys don't cry'.

Australian society's support and acceptance of traditional male behaviours can be seen in the advertising industry. The Solo drink advertisement showed a man in a dangerous exciting activity, rippling with muscles, wiping sweat from his brow, who drinks to quench a 'real' thirst — one assumes, of a 'real' man. The title of one surf life-saving contest is the 'Iron Man' competition. The use of the word 'iron' denotes strength, hardness, and durability, coupled with the image of 'man'.

Male and female social relationships are complicated by the fact that males and females have different ways of expressing themselves so they have difficulty understanding one another. Males have difficulty expressing their feelings, and indeed are encouraged not to express their feelings (Allen and Whateley, 1986; Radican, 1995; Rees et al., 1995). To a man, the way he shows a woman he loves her is by action — for example, by the sexual act — rather than by words. Work, to a man, is of primary importance, as it is his way of showing he cares for his family by providing money and goods for them. Protection of family is an important motivator of male behaviour and one way a man shows that he loves his family (Girvan, 1993). If a man is sick or injured he cannot provide for his family, therefore there is a tendency for men to deny emerging health problems.

MACHISMO AND HEALTH BEHAVIOURS

The need to appear masculine, not a 'sissy', influences men's health behaviours. Machismo is considered to be an element involved in male behaviour.

The differences between males and females are evident from early childhood. Boys have a greater frequency of accidents than girls (Jain, 1994), for example, falls from climbing, falls from skateboards and roller-blades, and bicycle accidents. The masculine stereotype behaviour of self-reliance in boys is reflected in the greater number of drownings and pedestrian accidents when compared to girls. Self-reliance would prevent boys from calling for help when in difficulties in the water, and would lead to boys being more independent in seeking play outside the home. There is also a strong element of risk-taking in these mortality statistics.

Risk-taking behaviour, aggression and dominance are implicated in the cause of certain health problems and mortality statistics. The major causes of death in males under the age of 24 years are accidents and suicide (Jain, 1994). Men are also twice as likely as women to die from car accidents (Jain, 1994).

After the age of 25 years men are most likely to die from cancer, cardiovascular disease and suicide (Jain, 1994). (Note that, in the majority of cases, nonbiological factors are important in the prevention of death from accidents, suicide and certain cardiovascular diseases.) Males of any age also suffer from a higher incidence of sporting injuries than women (Radican, 1995) It is common for males to 'play through' a sports injury, rather than leave the field or miss a game.

The characteristics of dominance and self-reliance lead to emotions being suppressed, contributing to the high incidence of mental illness and successful suicides amongst men. Machismo characteristics of stoicism, independence and lack of concern for personal health contribute to failure to seek help and support.

Stoicism and the fear of appearing weak or in any way feminine dominate male health behaviour (Fletcher, 1994; Radican, 1995; Saltonstall, 1993). The need to appear masculine in front of other men underlies many male behaviours. In an analysis of 296 taped visits by patients with a serious illness to their doctors (Pleck, 1995:18), male patients gave less information and asked fewer questions than female patients. However, men gave twice as much information to female doctors as they gave to male doctors. Men do not wish to appear 'weak' in front of other men.

Risk-taking behaviours and a lack of concern over the implications of these behaviours for their health contributes to men's increased rates of substance and alcohol abuse compared with women (Radican, 1995). By the age of 20 years, Australian men drink 10 times as much beer and 30 per cent more spirits than women (Smith, 1994). In the state of New South Wales, in 1992 (Fletcher, 1993), men were convicted of drink driving seven times more often than women. Head injury statistics from traffic accidents showed that five times as many men suffered from head injuries as women (Fletcher, 1993). It is suggested that such statistics are due, in part, to a combination of the following behaviours by male drivers:

- travelling at high speed;
- not wearing seat belts;
- not considering the weather or road conditions, e.g. rain and darkness; and
- driving whilst under the influence of alcohol.

The average life expectancy for an Australian male is six years less than that of a female (Grant and Lapsley, 1992). Not only do men die earlier but they are twice as likely to suffer from heart disease and have increased rates of most major illnesses compared with women (Grant and Lapsley, 1992; Ots, 1993; Radican, 1995).

The aggression and dominance of stereotypical masculine behaviour are reflected in the higher incidence of heart disease in men with Type A personalities compared with Type A women (Foreman, 1986:70; Helman, 1990; Myrtek and Greenlee, 1984). Type A behaviours are characterised by aggressiveness, ambition and competitiveness.

Most cancers are disproportionately represented in the male population (McKendrick, 1993:51). The following table (Table 2.1) shows the lifetime risk (0–74 years) of being diagnosed with a particular cancer, that is the morbidity risk. The mortality risk refers to the lifetime risk of dying from a particular cancer. The table illustrates the markedly increased risk of males dying from particular cancers compared with females.

Table 2.1 Comparison of male and female morbidity and mortality rates in commonly occurring cancers

Cancer	Sex	Morbidity risk	Mortality risk
Lung	M	1:18	1:21
	F	1:56	1:66
Melanoma	M	1:30	1:156
	F	1:42	1:368
Rectal	M	1:44	1:105
	F	1:85	1:210

(Compiled from statistics given in Coates et al., 1994)

Showing concern for one's health is not considered masculine (Foreman, 1986; Kron, 1995; Radican, 1995). This lack of concern results in men:

- being reluctant to visit doctors;
- taking fewer sick days off work when ill; and
- not seeking out health promotion programs or information.

Dr Gary Egger, who is involved with health promotion programs (Smith, 1994), described an incident in which he was lecturing to 100 navy men, and 10 per cent of the group discovered that they had symptoms of bowel cancer, prostate cancer or arthritis.

This lack of seeking help continues throughout life; older men have been found to access health services and social groups less often than women (*Better Health Briefing*, 1994). This lack of concern for health leads to a disregard or ignorance by men of the early signs of disease, leading to a higher mortality rate. In a study exploring health promotion in men (Fehir, 1988) participants filled in self-administered questionnaires on health, self-efficacy, lifestyle and health self-determinism. Those men who perceived themselves as having a high level of health and motivation for maintaining their health status still relied upon female partners to take partial responsibility for their health.

The nature of traditional male occupations also puts men at greater risk of serious accidents and illnesses than women (Ossler, 1986), for example,

- operating heavy machinery,
- undertaking heavy manual work,
- being exposed to hazardous chemicals and radiation, and
- working at 'dangerous' occupations such as firefighters and high-rise construction workers.

(Although some women are engaged in traditional male occupations, their numbers are small, and this is unlikely to change significantly.) The dangerous nature of some occupations appeals to the risk-taking nature of many men.

Men carry out about 90 per cent of violent crime (Biddulph, 1995) and 80 per cent of the victims of such crimes are men (Smith, 1994). These statistics reflect the machismo behaviours of aggression and dominance, and perhaps reveal a lack of ability to manage conflict situations other than through physical violence.

The statistics described are not unique to Australia. Worldwide, men's health is poorer than women's health. Men die younger, have a greater disease morbidity, seek help less often, and have higher rates of accidents and violent crimes compared with women (Allen and Whately, 1986; Arber and Lahelma, 1993; Forrester, 1986; Grant and Lapsley, 1992). An understanding of masculinity and machismo are needed in order to improve men's health.

MACHISMO AS A BARRIER TO HEALTH PROMOTION

Men consider they have more barriers to staying healthy than do women (Sommers et al., 1995). They have less time, they say, than women do to devote to their health and it's harder for them to get to a doctor. However, the major barrier to health promotion is men's lack of concern about their health and a disregard of the consequences of their behaviours and lifestyles.

Surveys have shown that even though men have more illness, disease and accidents than women, they engage in fewer health-promoting activities. Compared with women, men visit the doctor less often (Grant and Lapsley, 1992; ABS, 1995). Men also have fewer days off work and fewer work days of reduced activity, they take fewer medications and they visit a dentist less than often than do women (Grant and Lapsley, 1992). A recent survey (Kron, 1995) indicated that:

- 60 per cent of rural Australian men have never had a blood pressure check;
- 46 per cent have never had a skin cancer check; and
- 27 per cent have contemplated suicide at some time.

Some studies have sought to understand men's attitudes towards health. In a study of 'blue-collar' workers (Ritchie et al., 1991) it was found that men associated the behaviour of seeking better health as negative and thought it would result in a loss of individual control over their lifestyles. O'Connell (1989) found that the elements of knowledge, self-concept, and health beliefs were not influential in increasing men's frequency of testicular self-examination, however the behaviour of self-examination did increase. Similarly it was found that men were able to express their feelings in a men-only group (Rees et al., 1995). It is suggested, by the authors, that the men in these studies may have changed their health behaviour only when it was an agreed male group behaviour change — the desirable health behaviour was not exposing individuals to ridicule by other group members.

Public health screening and health promotion recommendations often target people who are in apparent good health. Men have been found to avoid seeking help when they are ill, so it is unlikely that they will actively engage in health-promoting activities based on the premise that they 'might' become ill. In one study, Sommers and others (1995) found that men exercising under doctors' 'orders' perceived themselves as more susceptible to illness than those who exercise of their own volition — 'I must be going to get sick if the doctor says I have to exercise to stay well!'.

Health promotion is a process of enabling people to increase control over, and improve, their health status (Tannahill, 1985). The major focus of health behaviour theories are the two concepts of **health-protecting (preventative)** and **health promoting** behaviours (Walker et al., 1987:76).

Health-promoting behaviours are directed towards optimising a person's sense of 'wellbeing' (Pender, 1987; Weitzel, 1989). Wellbeing is pursued because it is satisfying to the individual rather than a means to avoid disease. A study found that wellbeing in men is not associated with positive health behaviour (Ritchie et al., 1991). It is unlikely that men will appreciate the value of health promotion based on the avoidance of disease. Men do not, in general, actively engage in positive health behaviours.

Health-protecting behaviours describe the tendency of people to avoid situations where there is a probability of encountering illness (Walker et al., 1987:76). As we have seen already in this chapter, many men actively seek out situations where there is a high probability of illness or accident.

Using a health promotion model for men's health does not adequately address the motivational factors influencing male health behaviour. The health belief model put forward by Hochbaum and others (Becker, 1974; Rosenstock, 1974) is based on the theory that people will engage in certain health behaviours to avoid disease and illness. Evidence has been given that men do not engage in appropriate behaviours to avoid ill-health.

Traditional bases for health promotion and health belief theories do not address men's needs. A combined model is needed whereby men are encouraged to engage in health-promoting activities for reasons other than 'good' health. The motivating factors for men to achieve wellbeing need to be discovered and utilised when developing health promotion programs for men.

Even though machismo is a barrier to health promotion there is an increasing awareness by men that they suffer from poor health compared with women. Articles have appeared in the mass media addressing the issue of men's health (*Sunday Telegraph*, Sydney, 1994:117, 1995:37; Smith, 1994) as well as in popular health magazines (Fletcher, 1994; Radican, 1995), and in publications put out by some health insurance companies (Kron, 1995).

Male-initiated programs and support groups focus primarily on:

- urological problems,
- impotence, and
- divorce.

A cursory glance in the mass media shows advertisements for sexual health clinics dealing primarily with impotence. Some men have developed men's groups and support and information services via the Internet. Major issues of men's health that have direct impact upon men's mortality and morbidity are not addressed. Health promotion focusing on men's health is very sparse.

The focus on 'maleness' has been recognised as an important factor in successful health promotion programs (Fletcher, 1993; Kron, 1995; Ossler, 1986; Radican, 1995). A few programs have been successful in targeting some sections of the male population.

- The 'Gutbusters' program, initiated by Dr Gary Egger to decrease men's weight loss, focused on male vanity and not the health benefits of weight loss.
- In Sydney, the Greek community, concerned over the high incidence of smoking amongst Greek men, focused a program on the 'protective' nature of the male toward his family by questioning who would look after his family if he died.
- Apex clubs in Australia have held successful men-only groups to teach about and demonstrate testicular self-examination.

Another attempt to change male health behaviours was the introduction of a low-alcohol beer. The beer was not called 'light' but 'blue', focusing on men's avoidance of wishing to appear 'feminine' by noticeably following a healthier lifestyle. In another example, a health worker on an oil rig states that the men would not eat whole fresh fruit, yet would gladly eat fruit if it was peeled and cut for them (Smith, 1994). Health promotion programs can be effective if they focus on male motivational factors.

Successful men's health promotion is a challenge for all health professionals. Research into the motivating factors of men's health behaviours is difficult as men respond less to questionnaires than women do (Cox, 1985) and are less likely to reveal feelings in interviews (Pleck, 1995).

Women's health has become a political issue. Due to the strong pressure of lobby groups a National Women's Health Policy was launched in 1989. The policy aims to improve the health of Australian women, as well as directing the health system to be more responsive to women's needs (Townsend and McLennan, 1995). Men have no gender-specific policy for their health needs. It has been assumed that the current health system meets the health needs of men. Statistics and research have shown that this assumption is incorrect.

Expenditure on specific areas of men's health is far less than on women's health. Funding for research into prostate cancer in 1994 was 63 times less than research into breast cancer, although the death rates for both cancers are extremely similar (Smith, 1994:62). Part of the reason for this discrepancy is that it is often men who determine funding allocation, and there is a lack of interest by men in conducting research into men's health. Most men do not consider their health an issue. Health policies and strategies need to be identified, and supported, to enable the health system to be more responsive to men's health needs.

Characteristics of machismo and masculinity have been shown to have an adverse impact upon men's health. Many authors focus upon the negative aspects of masculinity. Authors have suggested that men should change their masculine behaviours and adopt more female behaviours. Androgyny, that is the expectation that men adopt some female characteristics, is a serious change for society as any change in men's expected behaviour would also cause a change in expected female behaviour. Men do not wish to become women and will resist any strategies that will make them appear more feminine. Health professionals cannot expect men to change their 'essential' self.

If we as health professionals decide to dampen or eradicate characteristic male behaviours then we, as a society, also lose the positive aspects of male behaviour. It is this very same aggressiveness, risk taking, dominance and self-assurance that led to the discovery and exploration of new worlds, and to continued scientific advances that have a major impact on our everyday lives. There is a need to direct masculine characteristic behaviours in a way that will have a positive impact upon men's health.

Health promotion programs need to be designed specifically for men. Some suggested strategies to be considered when developing health promotion programs for men are given below.

- Focus on characteristic male behaviours (e.g. male dominance, self-reliance, assertiveness, men-only groups) and utilise them in health promotion strategies.
- Focus on male motivators for health promotion, e.g. vanity, fear of appearing 'weak' or feminine.

- Encourage men to express their feelings in men-only groups.
- Educate male general practitioners (GPs) regarding men's health promotion.
- Use male GPs to encourage men to engage in positive health behaviours.
- Involve spouses/partners to encourage men's self-reliance in health.
- Lobby for funding for men's health issues and research.
- Provide easily accessible health programs for men, e.g. workplace health strategies.
- Lobby for political support in health policy development.

CONCLUSION

Men's health is poor compared with women's health. There is an increasing awareness by men and health professionals regarding the status of men's health. Strategies promoting positive health behaviours have been implemented with varying degrees of success. The most successful programs have been those that have recognised machismo or 'maleness' as important determinants of men's behaviour. Effective health promotion programs for men must seriously consider male behaviours as motivating factors in health activities. Through an understanding of male behaviour and 'machismo', barriers to health promotion programs can be overcome.

References

Australian Bureau of Statistics (1995): *National Health Survey: First Results*. Catalogue No4392.0. Canberra: ABS.

Allen DG and Whately M (1986): Nursing and men's health: some critical considerations. *Nursing Clinics of North America* 21 1: 3–13.

Arber S and Lahelma E (1993): Inequalities in women and men's ill-health: Britain and Finland compared. *Social Science and Medicine* 37 8: 1055–1068.

Becker MH (1974): *The Health Belief Model and Personal Health Behavior*. Thorofare, NJ: Charles B Slack. (25)

Bederman G (1995): *Manliness and Civilization*. Chicago: University of Chicago Press.

Bem SL (1981): Gender schema theory: a cognitive account of sex typing. *Psychological Review* 88 4: 354–364.

Better Health Briefing (1994): Men fare poorly in report on wellness 3 2: 31.

Biddulph S (1995): *Manhood: A Book about Setting Men Free*. Sydney: Finch.

Bilmes M (1992): Macho and shame. *International Forum of Psychoanalysis* 1 3–4: 163–168.

Boles J and Tatro C (1982): Androgeny. In: Solomon K and Levy NB: *Men in Transition: The Challenge of Change*. New York: Plenum Press, pp. 99–130.

Brannon R (1982): Inside the men's movement. *Ms* October: 40–44.

Coates M, McCredie M and Taylor R (1994): *Cancer in New South Wales Incidence and Mortality 1991*. Sydney: Cancer Council.

Connell RW (1995): *Masculinities*. Sydney: Allen and Unwin.

Cox CL (1985): The Health Self-Determinism Index. *Nursing Research* 34 3: 177–183.

Cunningham JD and Antwill JK (1980): A comparison among five masculinity–femininity–androgyny instruments and two methods of scoring androgyny. *Australian Psychologist* 15 3: 437–448.

Fehir JS (1988): Self-rated health status, self-efficacy, motivation, and selected demographics as determinants of health-promoting lifestyle behaviour in men 35 to 64 years old: a nursing investigation. PhD thesis. Austin, Texas: The University of Texas at Austin.

Fletcher R (1993): Men's Health Promotion: A Leading Role for Nurses? In: *Men's Health: The Forgotten Issue*. Melbourne, Australia: Ausmed Publications, pp. 1–8.

Fletcher R (1994): Blokes should have their own Ottawa Charter. *Better Health Briefing* 3 2: 16–17.

Foreman MD (1986): Cardiovascular disease: a men's health hazard. *Nursing Clinics of North America* 21 1: 65–73.

Forrester DA (1986): Myths of masculinity: impact upon men's health. *Nursing Clinics of North America* 21 1: 15–23.

Girvan Y (1993): The changing role of men in relationships. *Australian Association of Marriage and Family Counsellors* 45 July: 5–12.

Grant C and Lapsley HM (1992): *The Australian Health Care System*. Kensington, NSW: University of New South Wales, School of Health Administration.

Hargreaves DJ (1987): Psychological Theories of Sex-role Stereotyping. In Hargreaves DJ and Coolly AM (eds): *The Psychology of Sex Roles*. New York: Hemisphere, pp.27–44.

Harvey M (1993): Early sex-role socialisation in families. *Journal of Home Economics Association of Australia* XXV 4: 112–115.

Helman C (1990): *Culture, Health and Illness: An Introduction for Health Professionals*. Oxford: Butterworth Heinemann.

Hughes R (1987): *The Fatal Shore: A History of the Transportation of Convicts to Australia 1787–1868*. London: Collins.

Jain SK (1994): *Trends in Mortality by Causes of Death in Australia, the States and Territories during 1971–1992, and in Statistical Division and Subdivisions during 1991–1992*. Canberra: National Centre for Epidemiology and Population Health and Australian Bureau of Statistics.

Keisling BL, Gunther MD, Greene KS and Owen DL (1993): A behavioural self-report of masculinity: an alternative to trait, attitudinal, and 'behavioural' questionnaires. *Psychological Reports* 72 3 Pt 1: 835–842.

Kron J (1995): The men's healthcare debate. *MBF: Living Well* (Winter).

Leiner M (1994): *Sexual Politics in Cuba: Machismo, Homosexuality and AIDS*. Colorado: Westview Press.

The Macquarie Dictionary, 4th edn (1991). NSW: Macquarie Library.

McGrane T and Patience A (1993): Masculinity: Implications for Adolescent Sexuality in Australia. In: *Men's Health: The Forgotten Issue*. Melbourne, Australia: Ausmed Publications: pp 35–46.

McKendrick JJ (1993): Men's health: cancer. In: *Men's Health: The Forgotten Issue*. Melbourne, Australia: Ausmed Publications, pp. 47–53.

Moir A and Jessel D (1991): *Brainsex: The Real Difference Between Men and Women*. London: Mandarin.

Myrtek M and Greenlee MW (1984): Psychophysiology of type A behavior pattern: A critical analysis. *Journal of Psychosomatic Medicine* 26: 455–466.

O'Connell LG (1989): *The Influence of Knowledge, Self-concept, and Health Beliefs on Young Men's Practice of Testicular Self-examination*. The Catholic University of America: DNSC.

Orlofsky JL, Ramsden MW and Cohen RS (1982): Development of the revised sex role behavior scale. *Journal of Personality Assessment* 46: 632–638.

Ossler CC (1986): Men's work environment and health risks. *Nursing Clinics of North America* 21 1: 25–36.

Ots J (1993): Adam to A.D.A.M.: the social construction of men's health. In: *Men's Health: The Forgotten Issue*. Melbourne, Australia: Ausmed Publications, pp. 9–16.

The Oxford Dictionary (1990): Oxford: Oxford University Press.

Patience A (1990): Australia's hard culture: notes for an historical sociology. *Australian Studies* 14.

Pender NJ (1987): *Health Promotion in Nursing Practice* (2nd edn). Norwalk, CT: Appleton and Lange.

Pleck JE (1995): Gender Role Strain Paradigm: An Update. In Levant RE and Pollack WS (eds): *A New Psychology of Men.* New York, NY: Basicbooks.

Radican ND (1995): Helping men to help themselves. *The Essentials for Health and Fitness* 1 2: 32.

Rees C, Jones M and Scott T (1995): Exploring men's health in a men-only group. *Nursing Standard* 9 43: 38–40.

Richman J (1982): Men's Experience of Pregnancy and Childbirth. In McKee L and O'Brien M (eds): *The Father Figure.* London: Tavistock.

Ritchie J, Herscovitch F and Norfor J (1991): Beliefs of blue collar workers regarding coronary risk behaviours. *Newsletter: University of New South Wales School of Medical Education* 1 1: 1–2.

Rosenstock IM (1974): Historical origins of the health belief model. *Health Education Monographs* 2: 328–335.

Salonstall R (1993): Healthy bodies, social bodies: Men's and women's concepts and practices of health in everyday life. *Social Science Medicine* 36 7: 7–14.

Shapiro J (1992): *Men: A Translation for Women.* New York, NY: Dutton.

Smith R (1994): The gender trap. *Time (Australia)* 12 December: 56–60, 63.

Sommers JM, Andres FF and Price JH (1995): Perceptions of exercise of mall walkers utilizing the health belief model. *Journal of Health Education* 26 3: 158–166.

Sunday Telegraph (22 May 1994: 117): Health: strictly for men

Sunday Telegraph (5 February 1995: 37): Alarm as 'macho' men die of disease.

Tannahill A (1985): What is health promotion? *Health Education Journal* 44 4: 167–168.

Townsend K and McLennan W (1995): *Australian Women's Year Book 1995* Catalogue no. 4124.0. Canberra: ABS.

Villemez WJ and Touhey JC (1977): A measure of individual differences in sex stereotyping and sex discrimination: the 'macho' scale. *Psychological Reports* 41: 411–415.

Walker SN, Sechrist KR and Pender NJ (1987): The health-promoting lifestyle profile: development and psychometric characteristics. *Nursing Research* 36 2: 76–81.

Weitzel MH (1989): A test of the health promotion model with blue collar workers. *Nursing Research* 38 2: 99–104.

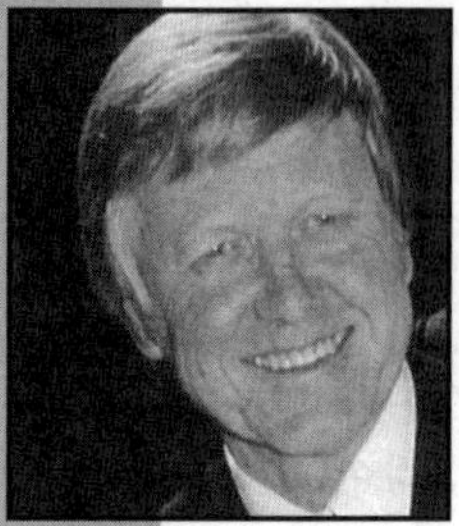

LEON EARLE

Bachelor of Arts, Master of Arts, Diploma of Teaching (Primary), Diploma of Speech and Drama, Master of Education, Doctor of Philosophy (Monash University)

Adjunct Associate Professor, Northern Territory University; Director, Earle Consultancy Services (Australia) and Earle Consultancy Services (Northern Territory)

As a gerontologist, Dr Leon Earle is highly respected both locally and internationally. He has provided policy advice to governments around the world and received awards for his programs, scholarship and professional addresses. Dr Earle has been responsible for the preservice, inservice and professional development training of thousands of people in the aged and human service fields in his role as a consultant, visiting international scholar and a member of the professional staff at both the University of South Australia and the Northern Territory University. Dr Earle was commissioned by the Minister of Ageing in South Australia to chair South Australia's Ten Year Plan on Aged Care Services and by the Minister of Health in the Northern Territory to prepare the Territory's Successful Ageing Vision Paper.

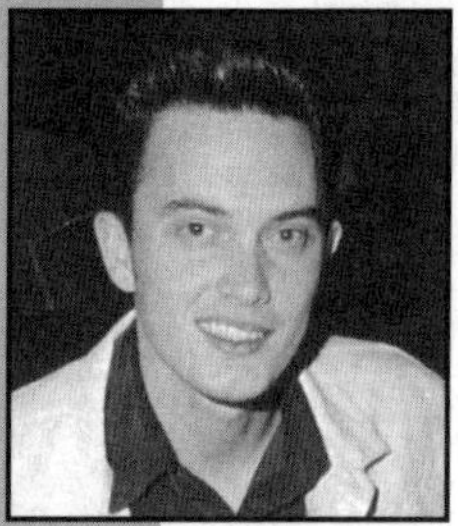

RICHARD EARLE

Bachelor of Arts

Media and Public Relations Coordinator, Earle Consultancy Services (Australia)

Richard Earle is a Bachelor of Arts graduate of the University of South Australia where he majored in media studies and community development (social policy) and completed a specialisation in communications. He has served as a university student president, branch director, activities officer, recreation officer, Media Relations Research Officer for Australia's National Seniors Association and a public relations coordinator in private and government sectors.

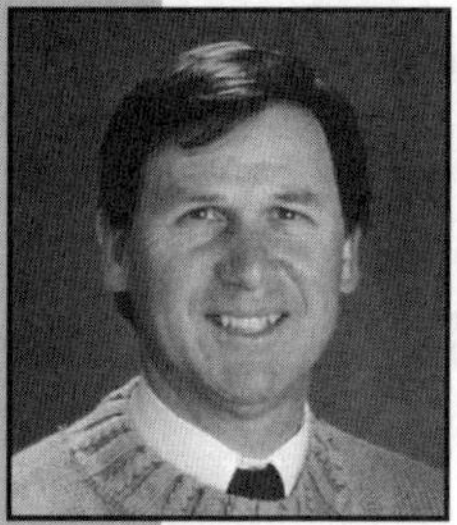

TONY EARLE

Bachelor of Education, Diploma of Teaching, Master of Education, Master of Psychology

Consultant, Earle Consultancy Services (Australia)

Tony Earle holds masters degrees in sociology (social psychology) and education (curriculum management) from the University of Missouri — Columbia, together with a Bachelor of Education and a Diploma of Teaching. His knowledge, speaking expertise and exceptional analytical skills have been sought locally and overseas by professional associations. His experiences include employment as a teacher, deputy principal and principal in schools, and as a university lecturer.

Chapter 3

Northern Territory men: Australia's social health and policy neglect

INTRODUCTION

The Northern Territory is a unique part of Australia. It is occupied by a people whose demographic composition and social profiles do not always fit conveniently into the centralist policies designed to meet the collective needs of those living in the somewhat different social context of generic urban Australia — more specifically, Canberra, Sydney, Melbourne and Brisbane.

In earlier decades, with its rugged frontier appeal, the Northern Territory attracted many resourceful people anxious to accept the range of challenges before them. Most of these were men. This is significant for two reasons:

1. The Northern Territory has more men than women.
2. It is the only Australian territory or state that has more men than women over 65 years of age.

It does not take much imagination to predict the carer (or, more correctly, lack of carer) implications for men without partners post-2000 and the associated professional health costs.

> **The Northern Territory enters the new millennium with Australia's youngest but most rapidly ageing population.**

The demographic and social context of the Northern Territory represents a crucial dilemma for policy and health professionals. The Northern Territory government has recognised the unique local needs and challenges. It seeks policies and programs for its people that are innovative, compensatory and need specific. At Federal government level however, funding and policies are designed to meet Australia's more generic needs. While these tend to be inclusive of the rest of Australia's states and the Australian Capital Territory, they do not meet the resourcing and servicing requirements of a population that is:

- remarkably geographically dispersed (11 large urban communities and 55 remote communities of 120–1000 people spread over a huge area);
- demographically unique (a comparatively young but rapidly ageing population with more men than women aged 65 years or more); and
- socially complex (an established multicultural population with the highest proportion of indigenous Australians — around 25 per cent).

Because the prevailing social context sets the scene for lifestyle patterns, an examination of the changing social context of the Northern Territory provides crucial indicators for the social living and health issues confronting male Territorians.

THE CHANGING SOCIAL CONTEXT OF TERRITORY LIVING

Economic growth and change

In the Northern Territory the social context has undergone significant changes during the last decade. These changes will influence the ways people live for the next 30 years. The nature and availability of work have changed with a shift from the primary (agriculture) and secondary (manufacturing) sectors to the tertiary (servicing) and quaternary (information processing) sectors. Tourism and trade have emerged as major industries across the Territory. By 2010 Darwin will offer not only a strategic location, but also an efficient world-class seaport connected to the national rail grid. With fewer males pursuing senior secondary and university education this represents decreasing employment opportunities for young males over the next decade which could translate into a negative impact on their social and mental health.

The Territory emerges as a place to stay

There is now evidence that more Territorians of all socioeconomic groupings intend to retire in the Territory, which has implications for accommodation, recreation, education, community activities and care services. Since 1995 more people have migrated into the Territory than out of it.

Changing values of the emerging aged

The current wave of Australians approaching the retirement years have had different experiences from their parents and will seek more diverse services in their retirement. In general they will:

- retire earlier,
- live longer,
- be more healthy,
- be more demanding and
- seek avenues for a long period of productive community involvement with full citizenship rights.

However, in the Northern Territory, many men will live their later years alone, lacking female partners — who tend to be pivotal in encouraging men to attend to their health needs.

Significant but narrowing differences between the Territory's cultural groups

The new millennium will herald significant but narrowing differences between the Australians of European, Asian and African descent (non-indigenous Australians) and Aborigines and Torres Strait Islanders (indigenous Australians). The characteristics of both groups are examined in Tables 3.1 and 3.2, with particular reference to life cycle trends.

The designation 'non-indigenous Australians' is used to represent people who do not have long-term (native heritage) links with the land. Non-indigenous Australians from non-English-speaking backgrounds comprise about 20 per cent of the population in the Northern Territory. Migration continues to boost numbers in this sector, which has implications for English proficiency needs. This is a crucial issue for men who are reluctant to visit health care professionals regularly. Not being able to communicate compounds the health problems.

During the 1990s permanent settler arrivals from neighbouring Southeast Asian countries exceeded 45 per cent of all the Territory's permanent settler arrivals, the highest proportion for any Australian state or territory. The family reunion line in Australia's migration program has given some migrants an avenue for bringing their parents to Australia. This will highlight variations between contemporary Australian family values among younger adult Australians and their aged parents.

In the case of older people of non-English-speaking backgrounds, many of those who have not become proficient in English have experienced adaptation difficulties (in the absence of work or other community participation forms) which have been linked to higher suicide rates. Moreover, many older migrants have experienced difficulties adapting to a changing social context that, for functional reasons, selects towards aged care in specialised residential complexes with professional support services rather than care in the home with mostly family and some community care program support. With more two-person working families featuring career women, increased lifestyle pressures and the need for personal recreation, professional care services at both ends of the life cycle continuum are becoming a more common necessity for many urban Territorians, including indigenous Australians. Post-2000 will see a greater dependency on child care and aged care services among indigenous and non-indigenous Australians, with the needs of indigenous Australians being for aged care especially. This pattern prompts consideration of a program whereby healthy older people, with or without grandchildren, might be given an opportunity to assist in the care and socialisation of young children in community or private settings, thus providing companionship for older Territorians.

The designation 'indigenous Australians' is used to represent people with long-term, native heritage links to the land. The life expectancy of indigenous Australians is lower than that of other Australians. While there have been many changes to the lives of contemporary indigenous people, the position of the aged reflects an enduring association with the land and kin. However, their access, role and status in some cases is now less assured within their communities, which has implications for their mental and physical health.

NON-INDIGENOUS AUSTRALIANS: CONTEMPORARYLIFE CYCLE FEATURES

Figure 3.1 Increased longevity over time among non-indigenous Australians (both descendants of post-settlement migrants born in Australia and migrants born overseas) in the Northern Territory

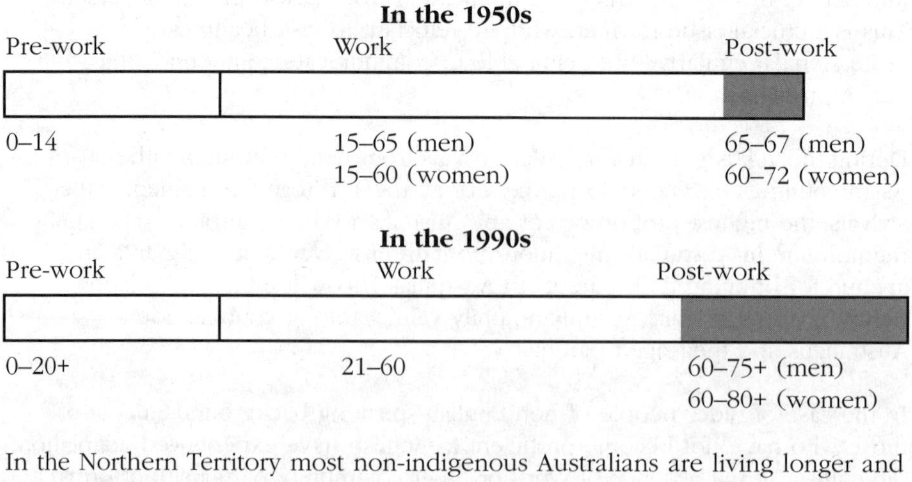

In the Northern Territory most non-indigenous Australians are living longer and retiring earlier. In the early 1950s, with a life expectancy of 67 years, men lived for about two years after retiring at 65, and women lived until about 72 years.

Today more men and women retire at 55–60 and live for another twenty to thirty years, which means that most Australians are 'younging' longer. In a sense many people are being given a 'third half' of living time! Planning ahead for this transition and the growing numbers of people involved is a crucial policy development challenge. Implicit in the changing social context and age profile of the Northern Territory are a number of new realities which must be considered in setting the scene for visionary policy development.

Selected life cycle features

- Young people stay at school longer, spending fewer years in the workforce and a longer period in the post-work years and therefore have less time to accumulate resources for retirement.
- The median age is projected to rise from about 35 years in 1998 to 42 years by 2050.
- The life expectancy of males is 75 years.
- The life expectancy of females is 81 years.
- Relocation of older people will become more prevalent with the rapid ageing of the population and community care expectations. Demand for home community care services will expand dramatically over the next decade.
- The emerging aged population in the Northern Territory incorporates a sizeable number of people who reveal symptoms of premature ageing (the hidden aged sector).
- The pending age wave will see 65-plus-year-old Territorians increase by about 75 per cent by 2006 (the year the first of the baby boomers reach 60). Nationally this increase will by about 19 per cent.

The implications of longevity for males is a major health issue because many lack the necessary preparation for retirement and therefore have ongoing activity and social interaction limitations. This sets the scene for subsequent social health complexities.

It is important that, at the Federal level, need-specific policies for Northern Territory people are supported. The rejection of the Northern Territory euthanasia legislation in 1997 highlighted gaps between Federal and local positions.

Post-2000 Reality 1

The Northern Territory has a rapidly emerging population of 'young aged' people who will live longer beyond retirement than ever before and in unprecedented numbers, and who will be seeking community involvement options outside work to maintain their sense of productivity and their social health.

INDIGENOUS AUSTRALIANS: CONTEMPORARY LIFE CYCLE FEATURES

While indigenous Territorians do not have the same life expectancy levels as the rest of the population, there have been important gains since the 1950s. Current life expectancy levels are around 55 for males and 62 for females. Standardised national death rates for indigenous Australians during the last decade have fallen from approximately 36 per 1000 to 26 per 1000. Because of the lack of demographic data on indigenous Australians until recently, it is more useful to highlight significant information across the life cycle of indigenous people during the 1990s and post-2000. While there is much to be done by the entire Australian community (indigenous and non-indigenous) to assist older indigenous people, the 1997 health promotion initiatives of the Northern Territory Health Minister Denis Burke, the ongoing sport programs and the crucial concession assistance measures for older people supported by Chief Minister Shane Stone, reflect an enduring commitment to encouraging positive community development.

Figure 3.2 Life cycle pattern among Northern Territory indigenous Australians

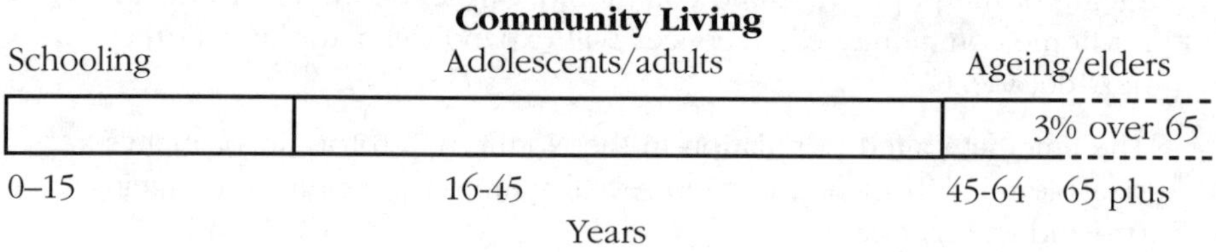

Selected life cycle features

- Indigenous Territorians make up around 25 per cent of the Northern Territory population (may be higher given the number of people not indicating whether they were indigenous or non-indigenous Australians at the 1996 census).
- Most leave school before they are 15 years old.
- Increasing numbers of indigenous students are entering higher tertiary education (e.g. at Northern Territory University 4.8 per cent of students are indigenous; Batchelor College provides specifically for indigenous students).
- The median age of the indigenous population is 21 years; the median age at death is 51 years.
- The life expectancy of Northern Territory indigenous males is 55 years (57 nationally).
- The life expectancy of Northern Territory indigenous females is 62 years (64 nationally).

- About 3 per cent of indigenous Australians live beyond 65 years.
- The nominated post-school community living years of 15 and over represent varying degrees of independence and dependence and this fact has implications for aged lifestyle needs.
- Older indigenous people tend to lack access to community support services and many are subject to abuse by some kin. This spawns health problems.
- There is a trend for increasing numbers of older indigenous people to live their more dependent aged years in specialised residential care centres.
- Relative to non-indigenous Australian males and females, indigenous Australian males are significantly less involved in work, education, community service and community recreation programs.

Post-2000 reality 2

The Northern Territory has an indigenous population, many of whom reflect the symptoms of ageing prematurely (relative to the rest of the population), who are in need of
- **family support,**
- **accessible/informed professional health services and**
- **the security of residential care.**

HEALTH ISSUES IMPLICIT IN THE NORTHERN TERRITORY'S SOCIAL CONTEXT

Personal responsibility for health

Both indigenous and non-indigenous older Australians will present planning challenges requiring collective community collaboration and coordination, as well as personal commitments from older individuals, to achieve a culture of social, mental and physical health. However, Northern Territory men will need to shift their attitudes to personal health care significantly. Tables 3.3 and 3.4 foreshadow the care needs post-2000 for the ageing Northern Territory population.

Post-2000 Reality 3

A major community development challenge for all older indigenous and non-indigenous Australians living in the Northern Territory is to take more responsibility for their personal health and social participation in the community.

Table 3.1 Northern Territory aged population: Projected increases beyond 1996 (percentages and numbers)

Age Group	1996-2001	1996-2006	1996-2011	1996-2020	1996-2031	1996-2051
45-64: No.	8000	15200	20300	22900	23900	33600
45-64: %	26	49	65	74	77	108
65 + No.	1700	4400	8500	25100	29300	37600
65+ %	29	75	144	425	497	637

(Based on ABS data)

Comments based on Table 3.1

The 45–64 age group will increase by approximately:

- 49 per cent over the next 10 years in the Northern Territory and 31 per cent nationally
- 74 per cent over the next 30 years in the Northern Territory and 28 per cent nationally
- 108 per cent over the next 50 years in the Northern Territory and 62 per cent nationally

The 65 plus age group will increase by approximately:

- 75 per cent over the next 10 years in the Northern Territory and 19 per cent nationally
- 425 per cent over the next 30 years in the Northern Territory and 106 per cent nationally
- 637 per cent over the next 50 years in the Northern Territory and 174 per cent nationally

Table 3.2 National and Northern Territory sex ratio projections
(Sex ratio is the number of males per 100 females)

Projected sex ratio data, 45–64 years and 65 years plus cohorts for the Northern Territory and nationally.							
Year	**1996**	**2001**	**2006**	**2011**	**2026**	**2031**	**2051**
NT 45–64	122.2	114.7	106.7	101.3	92.6	93.3	99.9
Aus 45–64	102.6	101.2	99.7	98.3	97.9	98.3	99.2
NT 65+	104.2	107.6	112.4	109.6	94.0	88.9	80.4
Aus 65+	77.1	78.5	80.9	82.7	83.2	82.0	79.3

(Based on ABS data)

Comments based on Table 3.2

- The Northern Territory has a higher sex ratio than the rest of Australia among 45–64-year-old people.
- The Northern Territory has a much higher sex ratio among people 65 plus.
- The Northern Territory and national sex ratio difference will be around 32 in 2006 among people over 65.

Given that, in the Australian community generally, women are three times as likely as men to be carers, the pending critical shortage of carers for a larger than usual male population in the Northern Territory will bring huge professional health costs unless strategies are introduced now to promote men's health.

National policies for 2006, based on a sex ratio of around 80 men to every 100 women, will ignore the needs of Territory men where the sex ratio will be around 112 men to every 100 women.

Productive community involvement needs for men

Earle (1996:62–66) has found that the issue of securing productive community involvement after retirement is most serious among men; the sector in surplus in the Territory. Without constructive and informed planning now, this issue will escalate and drain the professional health services dramatically. A long-term need is to provide boys with social and language skills programs in primary schools.

The hidden group of elderly — the Territory's 'old' young

Because the life expectancy of Aboriginal and Torres Strait Islander men is lower than any other sector in Australian society, policy planning for indigenous people must be age specific. Given that indigenous Australian men have a life expectancy of only 55 years, healthy lifestyle planning must become a feature of their lives. Many indigenous people in the 35–49-year age range have needs normally associated with people more than 60 years old. On a comparative basis only around 6 per cent of indigenous people are over 55 years, while the figure for the non-indigenous population is 20 per cent. The median age variation is around 13 years, with the non-indigenous figure at approximately 34 years and the indigenous figure at approximately 21 years.

Alcohol-related dementia is a serious issue in the Northern Territory. This adds significantly to the group of hidden elderly. Early dementia through substance abuse among both indigenous and non-indigenous males has emerged as an issue by placing strains on the already limited numbers of hostel and nursing home beds. The projected dementia increases for the Northern Territory between 1997 and 2011 will be around three times that of the national projections.

Innovative community involvement policies and programs must be developed for indigenous men in the Northern Territory to target three important issues:

- living standards,
- access to health services and facilities and
- the establishment of appealing activity programs to enhance community involvement prospects through recreation, education and community service initiatives.

Because of the unique social context of the Northern Territory, a vision paper to address challenges and needs for all older Territorians was initiated as a matter of priority by Health Minister, Hon Denis Burke, in 1997 (see Figure 8.2).

In the Northern Territory education remains a significant area of need for non-indigenous older people who are living longer and retiring earlier (or 'younging' longer) and also for indigenous people who have comparatively low life expectancy levels (or ageing earlier).

Given the somewhat transient nature of service providers (especially in rural/remote areas) and the unique social and health needs of Territorians, the challenges before health professionals are very demanding and must be recognised by the Federal government with respect to resourcing specific needs.

Specific policy and health care planning must include/consideration of:

- dementia levels in the Northern Territory increasing at a rate around three times higher than the national figure;
- the role of hospitals, which focus on acute care, in meeting expectations to service the diverse needs of older people;
- the relatively low profile given to aged care professionals;
- the already low levels of resources and projected needs;
- the delays in policy clarification;
- the diversity of varying cultural needs including indigenous peoples and their specific care requirements;
- accommodation needs and standards;
- coordination between and among the various sectors;
- training limitations/needs;
- the pressures (placements, finance, service provision) placed on staff in residential care centres; and also the other service provision sectors;
- cost efficiency and effectiveness in remote area servicing;
- a lack of range and flexibility in the national system;

- tensions caused by confusion (delays, terminology) and resource limitations in meeting needs (e.g. resident aggression);
- the illusion of research as a solution when the findings are often not put into practice at the doing level.

CONCLUSION

The policy challenge for Territorians post-2000 in meeting the needs of men will require a focus on:

- need-specific community development programs for those currently enjoying good health and
- initiatives for those in need of health care services who are more dependent upon residential programs.

Bibliography

Australian Bureau of Statistics (1997): *Census of Population and Housing, Selected Social and Housing Characteristics for Statistical Access Northern Territory.* Cat. no. 2015.7. Canberra: AGPS.

Australian Bureau of Statistics (1997): *Census of Population and Housing, Counts by Age and Sex for Selected Areas Northern Territory*. Cat. no. 2018.7. Canberra: AGPS.

Australian Bureau of Statistics (1997): *The Health and Welfare of Australian's Aboriginal and Torres Strait Islander Peoples.* Cat. no. 4704.0. Canberra: AGPS.

Australian Bureau of Statistics (1996): *Projections of the Population of Australian States and Territories 1995–2051*. Cat. no. 3222.0. Canberra: AGPS.

Australian Bureau of Statistics (1996): *Northern Territory in Focus 1996*. Cat. no. 1306.7. Canberra: AGPS.

Australian Bureau of Statistics (1996): *Australian Demographic Trends 1997*. Cat. no. 3102.0. Canberra: AGPS.

Australian Bureau of Statistics (1997): *Australian Social Trends 1997*. Cat. no. 4102. Canberra: AGPS.

Australian Bureau of Statistics: *Projection Series D 1987–2031*. Canberra: AGPS.

Earle L (1996): Successful Ageing in Australian Society: A Community Development Challenge. Adelaide: Recreation for Older Adults South Australia Inc.

Earle L and Earle R (1997): *Northern Territory Successful Ageing Vision Paper.* Darwin: ECS (NT).

Section Two

MEN'S HEALTH ON THE MOVE

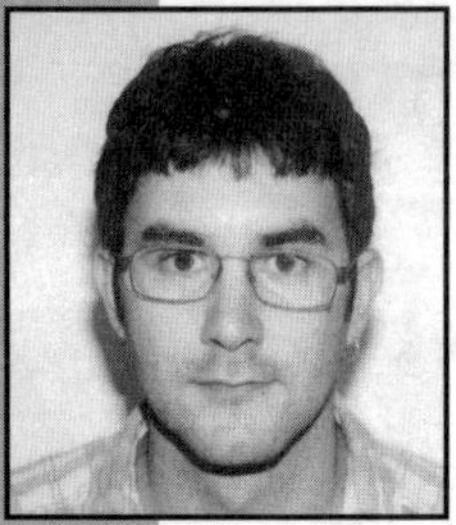

CHRISTOPHER ZIGURAS

Bachelor of Arts (Hons)

Curator, Human Mind and Body Program, Museum of Victoria, Melbourne

Prior to his current job Christoipher has lectured in the sociology of health at Griffith University in Queensland and worked as a writer of educational multimedia and video programs. He was a co-writer on the *SomaZone* adolescent health CD-ROM produced for the Victorian Department of Human Services, QUIT, Victoria Legal Aid and the National Asthma Campaign.

Christopher completed a Bachelor of Arts (Honours) at the University of Melbourne in 1992 and is currently completing a PhD in Politics at Monash University in Melbourne. His research deals with the popularity of self-help approaches to health care since the 1970s and explores the political dimensions of self-care in health. His most recent academic publication is 'The Technologization of the Sacred: Virtual Reality and the New Age' in David Holmes (ed.) *Virtual Politics: Identity and Community in Cyberspace*. London: Sage 1997.

Chapter Four

Masculinity and self-care

It has become commonplace to blame men's poor self-care for many of the health problems that men incur. Statistics would seem to indicate that men just cannot look after themselves. For example, we know that men:

- have higher rates of many preventable illnesses;
- use primary health care services less frequently; and
- have higher rates of most risk-taking behaviours [see chapters 1 and 2 in this book].

This chapter aims to shed light on the relationship between masculine cultures and health behaviour patterns as well as to identify social norms that have impeded improvements in men's health status. The following questions are a good indication of the problem and serve as a comparison to women's health and self-care behaviour:

- Why do men consume more tobacco, alcohol and illicit drugs?
- Why do men have more diet-related illnesses?
- Why do men die on the roads more often?
- Why do men often express themselves and problem solve through violence?
- Why don't men use health care services as often as women do?

To answer these questions, we must explore the concept of self-care and the ways in which men currently care for themselves.

WHAT IS SELF-CARE?

The concept of self-care can be separated into two categories — reactive and proactive.

Reactive self-care

People engage in reactive self-care when they are responding to an illness that has already developed. Reactive self-care usually involves:

- using some form of self-treatment;
- asking friends for advice; and, finally,
- seeking professional help.

Sometimes an identifiable condition provides a focus for action, sometimes there is merely a vague 'sick' feeling or a general malaise that prompts people to care for themselves more actively. Dean (1986) defines this type of self-care quite comprehensively:

> Self-care in illness is the range of individual behaviour involved in symptom recognition and evaluation, and in decisions regarding symptom responses, including decisions to do nothing about symptoms, to treat the symptoms by self-determined actions or to seek advice regarding treatment. Self-care thus includes consultation in the lay, professional and alternative care networks as well as evaluation of decisions regarding action based on the advice obtained in consultation (Dean, 1986:276).

The nursing profession has, in the past, promoted the concept of self-care primarily in the reactive sense. For example, Orem, who gave the concept of self-care a central position in her influential theory of nursing practice, orientated nursing practice around the patient's incapacity to provide the care they need because of their condition (Orem, 1991). The biomedical approach has also confined the patient's role in self-care to the reactive dimension. That is, doctors are primarily interested in a patient's responses to a specific disease and an appropriate cure. Moreover, the promotion of reactive self-care practices by our hospitals and other health agencies has created an emphasis on making the public aware of warning signs and symptoms of disease and encouraging people to get professional help early.

Men tend to engage in reactive self-care much later than women; self-treatment occurs much later in the course of illness, and less intensively than with women. Women visit general practitioners and alternative practitioners more often than men and take more medicines — prescription medicines, over-the-counter medicines and alternative medicines. A more specific example is the different rates of use of dental services by men and women. In Australia in 1996, 60.7 per cent of females aged 5 and over had a dental consultation compared with only 55.2 per cent of men of the same ages. However, of those who had a dental consultation, men (44.2 per cent) were more likely than women (38.9 per cent) to have had teeth filled (McLennan, 1997:201). The most plausible explanation for this is that males have dental checkups less often and delay visiting health professionals until their tooth decay is more advanced.

Proactive self-care

The second category, proactive self-care, encompasses all those everyday activities that people engage in to keep themselves healthy and to prevent disease. These include:

- eating a well-balanced diet;
- providing time for relaxing;
- paying attention to personal hygiene; and
- exercising.

Proactive self-care also involves avoiding known health risks, for example,

- drink driving;
- smoking; and
- engaging in unprotected sex.

Knowledge and skills related to self-care may be learnt at school or role modelled in the home by parents. Health care practitioners may inform and educate people in risk minimisation. For example, occupational health and safety nurses not only educate workers on the benefits of wearing safety equipment, they are also involved in organising safe systems of work and safe work environments. Public health policies in Australia have moved to emphasise the concept of proactive self-care by encouraging the avoidance of known risks to health and adopting a 'healthy lifestyle' approach. For example,

- the Slip Slop Slap campaign has been effective in reducing exposure to sunlight, the cause of most skin cancers; and
- using fluoride in public water supplies and toothpaste and encouraging regular brushing of teeth have reduced tooth decay problems in the community.

More informally, the producers of self-care products may advise their consumers to be proactive in self care.

In proactive self-care, men and women behave differently. This chapter will deal mainly with the relative lack of proactive self-care in men, and different approaches used to encourage men to actively maintain their own health.

ARE WE BLAMING THE VICTIMS?

In discussing self-care and health status, we must bear in mind that a person's health is more often affected by their social environment than it is by voluntary self-care behaviour (National Health Strategy, 1992). That is, the quality of the food supply, their working conditions, the level of air pollution and the life stresses men are subjected to affect their health just as much (if not more) than the health choices they make. Many of these variables are related to income levels. For example,

- cheaper housing is found near industrial areas and main roads but these tend to have higher levels of pollution than the tree-lined streets in leafy, more affluent suburbs; and
- the working conditions of blue-collar men are often more damaging to their health than the more cosy air-conditioned surrounds of men with white-collar jobs.

The distribution of wealth in Australia is very unequal and many studies have shown that wealth is one of the most important factors determining a person's health status (National Health Strategy, 1992). In short, higher levels of wealth and income translate into healthier choices.

Since the 1960s and 1970s it has become increasingly apparent that social and lifestyle factors are at least as important in determining the health of a population as the provision of health care services; governments around the world have set about trying to 'improve' the quality of life of their citizens (Dean and Kickbusch, 1995). However, the newfound interest in men's lifestyle has at times resulted in commentators blaming men themselves for their health problems. In a press release announcing the Australian Men's Health Conference held in Melbourne in August 1995, the then Health Minister, Carmen Lawrence, said,

> This conference will identify ways of targeting health promotion strategies to persuade men to take better care of their health and well-being (Vogel, 1995).

A number of papers at the conference focused on what Lawrence referred to as 'the behavioural issues that are having negative impacts on men's health', in particular dealing with drinking, dangerous driving and not seeking medical care (Vogel, 1995). While the Minister's comments may seem fairly inoffensive to most people, she has been criticised for 'victim-blaming', that is, blaming the victims for the state they are in, rather than focusing on the victims' circumstances. Peter Vogel stated that

> the suggestion that the poor state of men's health is their own fault was just below the surface of most of the promotion of the conference (Vogel 1995).

Vogel argues that, by looking at how individuals act without looking at the larger social issues which shape self-care behaviour, many at the conference gave the impression that men are simply lazy or careless. Vogel proposes instead that the men's health debate should focus on the broader social determinants of men's behaviour. According to Vogel, what is required is to

> . . . change models of masculinity, that is, to address all the social expectations that lead men to believe that to be a man means to behave self-destructively (Vogel 1995).

When discussing self-care it is important not to fall into overly 'individualistic' explanations that treat health behaviour as the free choice of the person, as if proactive self-care behaviour exists in a social vacuum. When we look at the cultural, social and economic influences on self-care we find that the self-care practices of individuals are influenced heavily by such factors as:

- the person's gender;
- their income;
- their level of education;
- their age;
- the place where they live;
- their ethnicity; and
- many other factors which are beyond the individual's direct control.

THE GENDER DIVISION OF 'CARING' WORK

Gender roles have perpetuated men's poor self-care and are a source of health inequality. To establish this point let us begin by looking at self-care as an integral part of lay health care. Lay health care is caring work which needs to be done in order to keep oneself, one's family members and one's friends healthy. As with other work, it is not distributed evenly between men and women (Dean, 1986). Despite changes in gender relations and family structures this century, women still carry out the vast majority of health care within the home (Eckerman, 1997). Women care for infants and children, for old and frail relatives, for sick or disabled family members and for men. Men have always relied on having women to look after their health. Not surprisingly, men who are in long-term relationships are generally healthier than single men and live longer (Lillard and Waite, 1995).

The gender division of lay care is part of the reason for women's higher rates of use of health care services. Because men on the whole work longer hours in paid employment, they find it harder to find the time to visit health professionals. Women on the other hand are more accustomed to seeking professional care because it is usually mothers who take care of children's visits to doctors and other health care practitioners.

A number of things have changed though, which leave men in a more vulnerable situation. On the one hand, heterosexual relationships have developed in a direction of greater mutual independence (Giddens, 1991); that is, women are becoming more demanding that men take care of themselves. In the not-so-distant past, most women were almost completely financially dependent on their husbands and fathers. The entry of women into the paid workforce has been driven in large part by their desire for greater economic independence. As a result, men are less able now to rely on a wife to perform those domestic duties on which their public lives rely, such as cooking, cleaning, caring for family members and so on. As Najman has observed,

> it could be argued that males now have less access to a loyal and caring servant (the wife); someone who has, at earlier times, been available to provide a wide variety of physical and emotional services (quoted in Dow, 1995).

It should be noted that it is still common for women to adopt a dual role by working in the paid workforce as well as doing the majority of the cooking, cleaning and caring but there is strong pressure on men to change since many women in this situation resent the domestic incompetence of their partners.

In this century, women's caring work has increasingly been taken over by agencies outside the family — by health care services, professional child care, psychotherapists and so on. At the same time, lay health care now is increasingly shaped by experts through self-help books, TV programs, magazines and advice from professionals. This popularity is not evenly spread, however, since self-help approaches have been taken up more readily by some social groups than by others; that is, by those with higher incomes and more education. Self-help has also been more popular with women than with men — women buy more self-help books, attend more support groups and buy more alternative health care products. From around the 1970s, many branches of health care practice entered a new phase, with a gradual shift in the way practitioners approach their public from seeing 'patients' as passive recipients of professional care (taking orders from the doctor) to encouraging their 'clients' to actively care for themselves. This professional shift has been accompanied by a broad grassroots movement to empower consumers of health care by giving people more control over their own health and patients more autonomy in relation to health care practitioners (Fox, 1988). Indicators of the grassroots movement include:

- self-help groups;
- the women's health movement;
- consumer rights movements; and
- the emergence of a wide array of alternative therapies.

In many instances, this interest in self-help was also taken up and encouraged by governments who saw a population caring for itself as an effective means both to improve the wellbeing of the citizens and to slow the rapidly increasing cost of curative health care services by redirecting resources to preventive measures. The popularity of these self-help approaches has been enormous, and has transformed the way we think about our health.

PROMOTING MEN'S SELF-CARE

In order to improve men's self-care there are two vital ingredients:

- the information about what to do and
- the motivation to do it.

Some men's self-care promotion deals with sex-related topics such as testicular self-examination, but more and more it deals with topics not related to male anatomy so much as to masculine lifestyles. These include anti-drink-driving campaigns or accident prevention in workplaces, both of which affect men far more than women. There is often debate about the merits of gender-specific health promotion for such issues. For example, in the case of suicide, where men's suicide rates far exceed women's, should suicide prevention campaigns approach men and women differently, placing special emphasis on young men, or should they ignore the gendered dimension of the problem? (Stewart, 1995)

The most basic self-care promotions targeted at men simply present information and assume that the audience are motivated to act on the advice. In the case of workplace accident prevention, this may take the form of a poster showing correct lifting techniques to avoid back injury. It seems that, on their own, these 'educational' approaches, which simply inform their audience, are not as effective as those which also motivate their audience to act on the information. The graphic nature of anti-drink-driving or anti-smoking television commercials released Australia-wide is intended to create an emotional impact (shock value) which has a much stronger effect than information alone. This is especially the case with men's health promotion, which has consistently faced the problem that many men do not want to be seen to care too much about their own vulnerability.

Even when men make healthy choices they are often embarrassed about their healthy behaviour in front of other men. Take the example of Tooheys strategy in marketing light beer to men. Men drink far more beer than women, 10 times as much by one estimate (Smith, 1994). The promotion of low-alcohol beer by the beer companies was not so much a response to health concerns as a means of retaining the volume of beer sales after the introduction of random breath testing in most states in the 1980s. Tooheys was the most successful of the brewers in pushing light beer, by drawing attention away from health concerns, which they figured would make men feel wimpy. 'We knew that men were reluctant to be heard ordering a light beer,' Paul Czerny, marketing manager of Tooheys, told *Time* magazine. 'It just seemed wimpy; but by leaving out the word "light" and calling the product "Blue", nobody would feel inhibited ordering one in front of their mates.' This strategy worked remarkably well and facilitated a move from heavy to light beer, rather ironically by ignoring light beer's health benefits.' As Czerny explains, 'The idea is not to focus on health and safety worries, but to find something men can relate to.' (Smith, 1994:60).

There is a common argument that it is masculinity which is the problem with men, that is, men's culture and behaviour are the root cause of many of their health concerns. Norman Dean Rodican, a men's health educator at Sydney's Royal North Shore Hospital, argues that, 'if we are going to do anything about the appalling state of men's health, we really have to redefine our concept of masculinity.' (Smith, 1994: 61) This perspective is increasingly put forward in policy discussions surrounding men's health promotion. However, the suggestion that masculine identity in its entirety needs overhauling presents health workers with a daunting task. Is the public health care system capable of launching a whole new sphere of social engineering which is directed at shifting men's image of themselves away from one type of masculinity and replacing it with a 'healthier' male culture? This is a big crusade to embark on, but many men's health advocates have proposed this type of cultural shift without seeming to be aware of the enormity of the task they are proposing. This is compounded by the fact that, while the women's movement was propelled by a popular sense of inequality and injustice, in stark contrast, the men who are most at risk don't actually seem to want to change themselves or the society they live in to any significant degree. This factor retards any move toward improvements in the level of proactive self-care.

From an early age, boys are 'toughened up'. This is a central feature of the dominant form of Australian masculinity and a characteristic of Australian men which impacts seriously on their health. Boys are taught to enjoy the gruelling regimes shouted at them by coaches on the football fields of Australia. They are taught to tolerate pain and physical suffering because it is a sign of strength. Boys are taught to equate vulnerability and weakness with femininity and homosexuality. It is important to remember that the toughness of Australian masculinity is defined in opposition to two groups who are considered inferior — women and homosexual men. The body in this dominant masculine culture is not to be enjoyed for its own sake but is to be toughened up for use in the organised aggression of the sports field (Webb, 1991–2, 1995). While girls are encouraged to be communicative and sociable from an early age, boys are encouraged into managed competition with each other. In the process, Coward observes,

> men not only lose contact with that part of themselves that wants to take care but they also find it difficult to ask for care. They become set on paths of isolation, distant from each other and emotionally dependent on women (Coward, 1987: 14).

Let's consider what men gain from disregarding their health. Health workers have to realise that good health is not everyone's highest priority and that, in some cases, men may actually benefit from neglecting their own self-care. The physical and emotional stresses which some men put themselves under can have payoffs if they are willing to do the most dangerous jobs, work the longest hours and so on. It is no surprise that women who follow some of the more gruelling, traditionally male career paths also develop the health complaints that men in those positions do. More importantly though, men's abrogation of responsibility for caring work (in that they spend less time caring for themselves, their families and their friends) means that men have been able to achieve positions of power in the paid workforce by virtue of having women to look after them and their families. The men's movement has often portrayed men as the victims of a system which denies men's nurturing role. The nurturing role is very closely linked to proactive self-care behaviours. It is undeniable though that men have benefited in the paid workforce from the unpaid caring work which women do. The traditional division of labour has involved a trade-off for men in which a loss of direct family contact has been compensated for by men's power in the paid workforce. Prominent Australian feminist author Eva Cox is dismissive of the men's health movement for this reason. She told *Time* magazine:

> Frankly, men have wielded all the power for years and if they don't like the situation, they've got only themselves to blame. You don't see any men stepping down from power because it may affect their health. I'd gladly be the head of BHP and risk losing a few years off my life expectancy, but I doubt if the head of BHP would be willing to swap (Smith, 1994: 60).

The problem with this argument is that Cox portrays all men as sharing the same situation. While it is true that some men who conform to the dominant form of masculinity are rewarded with power, prestige and wealth, most men, like most women, are not heads of multinational corporations. Some men may be rewarded for neglecting their health by climbing the career ladder faster and earning higher incomes than men who have a more rounded life. In this case they are relying on reactive self-care. For most men, though, the sacrifices are made not for personal rewards but out of economic necessity. Historically, most men have worked in relatively dangerous occupations in agriculture and manufacturing and have been raised with the ethos that they must sacrifice their own health to earn income to support their family. The proportion of men who work in such blue-collar occupations is decreasing but the culture of physical work remains strong. One of the reasons that men with low income and education levels have a poorer health status is because they must often settle for the dirtiest and most dangerous jobs. In this way they are forced to rely on reactive self-care, on health agencies providing support during illness. In stark contrast to the image of the stressed executive making sacrifices for the sake of his career, it is often the lowest paid and most unpleasant jobs that have the worst effects on men's health.

THE WAY MEN VIEW THEIR BODIES

Given this culture, how can men's health promotion encourage men to respect their bodies more and be proud of looking after themselves and others rather than being embarrassed? As we've seen from Tooheys strategy, one approach is to disguise the healthy behaviour so it does not appear 'wimpy', but this is a temporary solution which does not tackle the fundamental problem that, in the dominant culture, worrying about one's health is seen as a sign of weakness.

One approach is to tap into the fact that, in recent decades, physical appearance has become more important to Australian men. This is perhaps partly due to the increased representation of well-built and well-groomed men in film, television and magazines. Advertisers increasingly use images of attractive men to sell products to both men and women. Men's appearance is also becoming increasingly important in the workplace. This is most obviously the case in service industries, such as hospitality, retail and entertainment, where workers have a high level of customer contact. As with the media, employers believe that the public does not want to look at messy and unhealthy men. For middle-class and professional men, being seen to be able to take care of one's own health is seen as an indication of personal mastery and self-control, whereas being overweight or having an unkempt appearance is taken as a sign of a lack of self-control or a lack of willpower. Echoing this concern, Bruce Marshall, a partner at accounting firm KPMG, who works in executive personnel placement, told *The Bulletin* magazine that it was becoming more difficult to find positions for overweight executives:

> 'In organisations which feel the need to be trim, taut and terrific', he observed, 'an overweight executive is out of place.' (Bagnall, 1996: 18)

Large organisations are becoming increasingly conscious of the relationship between their employees' productivity and their health. This class-related dimension of masculine proactive self-care is apparent in statistics on self-care behaviour for men which show that men with higher incomes or more education are generally more active in pursuing positive self-care behaviours (Turrell, 1995). These are also the men with high disposable incomes who are targeted by companies who sell men's health products, such as gyms, sports suppliers, and magazine publishers.

One of the first men's health promotion campaigns to appeal to men's consciousness of their physical appearance was, perhaps not surprisingly, a weight loss program designed specifically for men. The Gutbusters male weight loss program was developed by Gary Egger, who researched the program by talking to men in the Newcastle Steelworks about their beer bellies. This approach focused on men's body image in order to change their eating and exercise patterns. Talking to overweight men Egger found that,

> telling men they should worry about diet and blood pressure will get you nowhere. But all men want to look good, and once you get rid of the pot belly you're well on your way to solving heart, diet and blood pressure problems as well (quoted in Smith, 1994:60; see also Kennedy, 1995).

In cases like this, we can see some positive progress in encouraging men to engage more actively in proactive self-care practices. Campaigns like Gutbusters are successful because they are culturally appropriate; that is, they understand the men they are communicating with and they understand the social environments in which their audience lives. It is important to remember that, as Australia is a culturally diverse society, there are very different forms of masculinity existing alongside one another. Approaches that work for one group of men will not necessarily work for others. To illustrate this point, consider the way cooking pages are presented in two new Australian men's magazines. The ability to cook for oneself is a fundamental aspect of being able to manage one's diet and care for dependent others. The first issue of *Ralph*, a magazine which tries to appeal to 'Aussie blokes' introduces its cooking pages thus:

> Men of Australia, liberation is at hand! For too long we've been reduced to dependent status in the kitchen, where the simple pleasure of preparing a

> decent feed has been denied us by cruel, insensitive women. To cook for yourself is to be free! And girls think it's sexy. Let's rock (Ralph, 1997:114).

There is an embarrassed tone associated with cooking in *Ralph*. There is no mention of healthy eating but plenty of sexual overtones and beer swilling in the kitchen. It is aimed at men who are not interested in cooking but would cook to impress a girl. At the other end of the spectrum, another new magazine, *Men's Health*, takes a very different approach. Cooking is introduced in a very different way, to a very different audience:

> You've just finished a work-out, a long ride or one too many drinks after work. You don't want to mess up your system with a greasy take-away, but you're hungry — now. What's a man to do? Try these simple, delicious recipes to fill that gnawing void in your life (*Men's Health*, 1997).

What follows are four pages of recipes to satisfy hunger quickly and healthily. The target reader is a white-collar worker who exercises regularly but likes to party sometimes. The recipes are suggestions about what to eat when 'you come home from the gym'. . . 'you're coming down with the no lunch syndrome' . . . 'you've finished 100 km on the bike'. . . and 'you tumble home after Friday night drinks'. As we can see, there are very different masculine cultures of self-care, even when it comes to a task as fundamental as preparing food. However, masculinity works towards proactive self-care in these examples.

These examples from men's magazines provide some insight into the cultural differences which operate between men from different social classes and which influence the fact that men with higher incomes and higher levels of education engage in more positive self-care behaviour. While socially disadvantaged groups make equal use of curative health care services, and more use of medical services, they

> use health promotion and disease prevention services at a significantly lower rate than more advantaged groups (National Health Strategy, 1992:109).

And to understand why that is, it is necessary to view these different cultures (blue-collar 'blokes' as opposed to white-collar 'yuppies') in light of their material living conditions. Blue-collar workers and poor men are reminded daily that physical sacrifice is a necessary part of life — their work is dirtier and involves more risk of accidents, their suburbs are more polluted, their old cars are more dangerous — and so they are forced to put health lower down on their list of priorities. Wealthier men can avoid many of these health risks. In addition, for better-off men, health and wellbeing is becoming a marker of social status. If labouring men traditionally thought of their bodies as a tool, the new health-conscious middle-class men think of their bodies as a work of art. For the readers of *Ralph* the body is something you use for work, and which is worn out by work. For the readers of *Men's Health*, who work with their brains and play with their bodies, physical enjoyment and positive health are ends in themselves. And as the gap between rich and poor gets bigger in Australia, so too does this cultural gap in the way men treat their bodies.

CONCLUSION

It is pointless trying to change masculinity as a whole; it is pointless to blame individual men for not looking after their own self-care. In trying to promote positive self-care to men we need to understand the ways men think of their bodies and how this is related to their lives more broadly. Health promotion messages for men need to be very attuned to the cultural diversity of Australian men in the 1990s.

References

Bagnall D (1996): Beauty and the beasts. *The Bulletin*. 29 October: 16–19.

Coward R (1987): High time men changed. *New Internationalist* September: 13–14.

Dean K (1986): Lay care in illness. *Social Science and Medicine* 22: 275–84.

Dean K and Kickbusch I (1995): Health-related behavior in health promotion: Utilizing the concept of self care. *Health Promotion International* 10 1: 35–40.

Dow S (1995): What does the case of Shaka Manna mean for men's mental health? *Age*. 10 June, p.18

Eckerman (1997): Women as carers: the importance of context. Paper to the Chronic Illness Alliance Conference. Melbourne. 28 April.

Egger G (1994): Male obesity and the Gut Buster program. *Health Issues* No. 41 December: 31–32.

Fox R (1988): The medicalization and demedicalization of American society. In: *Essays in Medical Sociology: Journeys in to the Field*. New Brunswick, NJ: Transaction Books, pp. 465–83.

Giddens A (1991): *Modernity and Self-Identity: Self and Society in the Late Modern Age*. Cambridge: Polity Press.

Kennedy F (1995): Big on guts: a new image for the all-Aussie male. *The Weekend Australian* 30 September–1 October: 3.

Lillard LA and Waite LJ (1995): 'Til death do us part: Marital disruption and mortality. *American Journal of Sociology*. 100 5: 1131–1156.

Men's Health (1997): What to eat when. *Men's Health* (Australia). October Issue 1: 82–5.

McLennan W (1997): *1997 Year Book Australia*. Canberra: Australian Bureau of Statistics.

National Health Strategy (1992): *Enough To Make You Sick: How Income and Environment Affect Health*. Canberra: National Health Strategy.

Orem D (1991): *Nursing: Concepts of Practice* (4th edn). New York: McGraw Hill.

Ralph (1997): Tucker. *Ralph: Secret Men's Business*. August: 114–5.

Smith R (1994): The gender trap. *Time*. 12 December: 56–61.

Stewart M (1995): Young male suicide — reversing the trend. *XY: Men, Sex, Politics* 5 1.

Turrell G (1995): Social Class and Health: A Summary of the Overseas and Australian Evidence. In: Lupton GM and Najman JM (eds) *Sociology of Health and Illness: Australian Readings* (2nd edn). St Lucia: University of Queensland Press, pp. 113–142.

Vogel P (1995): Dying to be noticed. *Certified Male*. Summer.

Suggested reading

Altman D (1987): The myth of mateship. *Meanjin* 46 2: 163–172.

Australian Men's Health Network (1997): The relative importance of men's and women's health. *AMHN Newsletter* 7: 2–3.

Australian Men's Health Network (1997): The evidence for discrimination against men. *AMHN Newsletter.* 7: 4–5.

Biddulph S (1995): *Manhood: An Action Plan for Changing Men's Lives* (2nd edn). Sydney: Finch Publishing.

Boston Women's Health Book Collective (1971): *Our Bodies, Ourselves: A Book By and For Women*. New York: Simon and Schuster.

Broom D (1995): Masculine Medicine, Feminine Illness: Gender and Health. In: Lupton G, Najman J (eds): *Sociology of Health and Illness: Australian Readings* (2nd edn). South Melbourne: Macmillan.

Commonwealth Department of Human Services and Health (1995): *Draft National Men's Health Policy*. Canberra: Australian Government Publishing Service.

Connell RW (1987): *Gender and Power: Society, the Person and Sexual Politics*. Sydney: Allen and Unwin.

Connell RW (1991): Live fast and die young: the construction of masculinity among young working-class men on the margin of the labour market. *Australian and New Zealand Journal of Sociology*. 27 2: 141–71.

Connell RW (1996): The politics of changing men. *Arena*. No. 6: 53–74.

Fay S (1996): Men's health policy. *Health Issues* 46: 34–5.

Hewitt N, Elliot B, Shanahan P (1995): *A Review of Risk Behaviours Among 15–24 Year Olds*. Canberra: Commonwealth Department of Human Services and Health.

Jenkins P (1991): 'I'm fine, really': Why are men conspicuous by their absence from the doctor's waiting room? *Achilles Heel: The Radical Men's Magazine,* Issue 11, Summer.

Kickbusch I (1989): Self-care in health promotion. *Social Science and Medicine* 29 2: 125–30.

Ozanne T, Schliemann G, Zask A, North G, Beaty S and Curran P (1996): Men on the line: a survey of telephone referral and counselling services for men. *Certified Male*. Winter.

Pearson A (ed.) (1993): *Men's Health: The Forgotten Issue*. Melbourne: Ausmed Publications.

Pease B (1991): Changing the Story for Men: Mythopoetic and Sociological Perspectives. In: Frank L (ed.): *Changing the Story*. Proceedings of the 1991 National Women and Drugs Conference, University of Melbourne. Melbourne: Addiction Resource Institute of Victoria.

Riehl-Sisca J (1985): Orem's general theory of nursing: an interpretation. In: Riehl-Sisca J (ed.): *The Science and Art of Self-Care*. Norwalk, Connecticut: Appleton-Century-Crofts.

Sabo D and Gordon F (eds) (1995): *Men's Health and Illness: Gender, Power and the Body*. Thousand Oaks, California: Sage.

Steiger NJ and Lipson JG (1985): *Self-Care Nursing: Theory and Practice*. Bowie, Maryland: Brady Communications.

Verbrugge LM (1985): Gender and health: An update on hypotheses and evidence. *Journal of Health and Social Behavior* 26: 156–82.

VicHealth (1996): Young people's health. *VicHealth Letter: The Victorian Health Promotion Foundation Newsletter* 4: 3–5, 14.

VicHealth (1997): Men's and women's health. *VicHealth Letter: The Victorian Health Promotion Foundation Newsletter* 6: 3–14.

Webb J (1992–3): In the flesh. *XY: Men, Sex, Politics* 2 4 Summer.

Webb J (1995): Doing ourselves an injury. *XY: Men, Sex, Politics*. 5 3.

White R (1997): Young men, violence and social health. *Youth Studies Australia* March: 31–7.

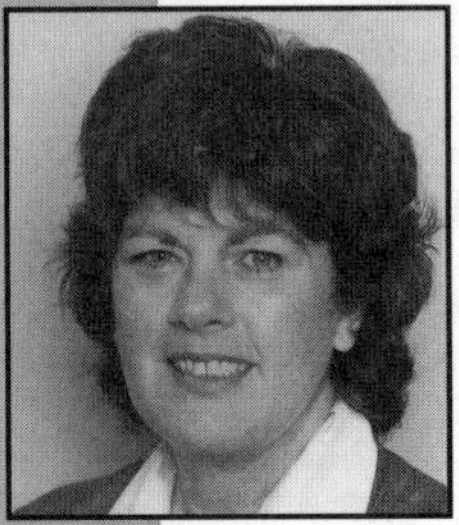

CHARLOTTE DE CRESPIGNY

Registered Nurse, Bachelor of Nursing, Graduate Diploma in Primary Health Care, Fellow of the Royal College of Nursing, Australia
Lecturer in the undergraduate nursing program at The Flinders University of South Australia

Charlotte has worked as a clinician and educator in the drug and alcohol field for 10 years. She recently established, and now coordinates, the national postgraduate alcohol/drug nursing studies program in the School of Nursing at The Flinders University of South Australia. She is also attached to the National Centre for Education and Training on Addiction (NCETA). She is a doctoral candidate with Flinders and NECTA. Her doctoral research is into young women's social drinking and environments but she is involved in other research on older women and medication use, and the clinical learning of mental health undergraduate nurses. She provides staff development and consultations to services on matters related to primary health care and alcohol and drug use.

Chapter 5

Alcohol and other drug use issues in contemporary Australia

INTRODUCTION

The aim of this chapter is to provide the reader with an overview of alcohol and other drug use in Australia, and to present the relationship alcohol and other drug use has to men's health. Some commonly used substances and related issues are discussed; however the major emphasis is on alcohol due to its high level of use and its related problems amongst men in the Australian community.

THE SOCIAL AND ECONOMIC COST OF DRUGS

In 1992, the impact of alcohol problems on the Australian economy totalled more than $4.4 billion or 24 per cent of all drug-use costs (Collins and Lapsley, 1996). In each year many young men die or are severely injured through accidental injury associated with hazardous alcohol consumption.

Three-quarters of all drug-related deaths in Australia are from smoking (Single and Rohl, 1997; English et al., 1995). In 1992 the economic costs of tobacco use were estimated at about $12.7 billion or 67.3 per cent of the total cost of all drug-related costs (Collins and Lapsley, 1996). Males are three times more likely than females to die from tobacco-related causes (Single and Rohl, 1997).

Those who die as the result of illicit drug use tend to be young. On average each death results in 36.7 years of potential life lost (compared with 4.7 years of potential life lost through death from tobacco-related causes) (English et al., 1995). Deaths from illicit drug use are preventable in the majority of cases and are most often related to impurities and unknown doses of the drugs used. Poly-drug use is commonly implicated in a significant number of accidental deaths (sometimes described as overdoses) amongst casual and regular users. Death often results through the combined use of more than one substance, for example, alcohol, heroin and prescription drugs such as sedatives (Hall, 1996).

Up until the middle of 1995 a significant number of young men and women who injected illicit drugs are known to have contracted HIV infection through their injecting drug use. The numbers were disproportionately biased towards men (940) compared with women (186). This is a major concern for men's health (Single and Rohl, 1997).

ALCOHOL

Alcohol is a central nervous system depressant. It slows thought processes and body functions, especially in large doses, and the user can overdose if excessive amounts are used.

In Australia about 76 per cent of the adult Australian population consumes alcohol — 80 per cent of men and 72 per cent of women. Frequency of drinking is more evident in men than in women (Single and Rohl, 1997).

Recent Australian figures on unsafe levels of alcohol consumption show that 16 per cent of adolescent males binge drink, that is they consume seven standard drinks or more in one weekly session. Only 5 per cent of adult males binge drink. About 13 per cent of men and 23 per cent of adolescent males are 'heavy' drinkers (more than seven standard drinks a day for at least 2 days a week) (Single and Rohl, 1997). Young men between the ages of 16 and 24 years are at most risk of alcohol-related harm in the male population (National Drug Strategy, 1995).

There is growing evidence that men who drink at light-to-moderate levels (between two and four standard drinks a day) have a reduced risk of coronary heart disease (Fuchs et al., 1995) and gallstones (Pols and Hawks, 1992). However, men who are harmful drinkers (more than four standard drinks a day) are at risk of developing alcohol-related health problems due to their excessive, regular and hazardous alcohol consumption.

In 1992 the National Health and Medical Research Council reported that at least one in five hospital admissions is due to alcohol-related injury, and hospital records and morbidity and mortality data attest that illnesses such as cancer (of the neck and throat), and heart, stomach and liver disease have been common features of adult male ill-health (Pols and Hawks, 1992; Single and Rohl, 1997). In 1995, twice as many Australian males as females died as a result of alcohol-related liver damage, cardiac problems, cancers and gastrointestinal problems. More males than females reported memory dysfunction or loss associated with drinking.

Spectrum of alcohol problems

Significant numbers of young people (mostly males) die each year from car accidents. One-third of all driver fatalities have blood alcohol levels (BALs) over the legal limit of 0.05 BAL, and 70 per cent of those are over 0.15 BAL (NDS,1995). Other problems associated with intoxication include verbal and physical assaults, domestic injuries and work-related accidents. Alcohol is a significant factor in many drownings. Being a perpetrator or victim of crime is also likely to stem from a combination of alcohol and interpersonal problems (Single and Rohl, 1997).

As with other drugs which affect the central nervous system, regular excessive consumption of alcohol results in neuro-adaptation. The neuro-adaptation process, alcohol-related liver disease, pancreatitis and the Wernicke-Korsakoff syndrome have each been related to genetic factors by various researchers. The relative contributions of heredity and environment to these conditions are uncertain (Pols and Hawks, 1992) and caution is needed in making any claims of genetic links with alcohol (or other drug) problems.

The least common alcohol-related problem is dependence, with only about 10 per cent of drinkers being affected. Alcohol dependence occurs when alcohol is used daily in excessive doses over at least several weeks. Neuro-adaptation occurs when the central nervous system adapts to the pharmacological effects of alcohol. Such tolerance can then occur to a level where the drinker no longer experiences the intoxicating effects of the substance. The drinker then needs to use increased regular doses of the drug to feel normal. Drinkers will experience withdrawal symptoms when the substance is ceased. In severe cases, withdrawal symptoms will occur when the blood alcohol level drops significantly.

Alcohol dependence usually results from a combination of psychological, environmental and alcohol effects impacting on the drinker. The excessive daily use of alcohol is usually an attempt to cope with or respond to complex life problems. For some people addiction occurs at the time of a life crisis or a stage in their personal development. These may be times of psychological pain, unresolved grief and loss, loneliness, cultural distress and dislocation, or other life changes such as loss of job, partner or home. Drinking heavily at these times may ease the emotional pain.

Alcohol and heroes

Although the facts just presented are almost common knowledge in the community, there is no shortage of customers for alcohol as a popular commodity. An aspect of this phenomenon may lie in the relationship between alcohol and masculinity, as epitomised in and by sporting sponsorship and role models who drink in public.

Alcohol has been, and still is an important icon in Australian male culture. Beer has played an enormous role in men's socialising and mateship and in their social health problems when it is used at harmful levels.

Public education about safe drinking can be undermined easily by irresponsible alcohol marketing which portrays men in hazardous drinking situations. An example of such marketing was shown recently on commercial television. A group of hard-working, fit-looking men were at the end of a long day's work in a hot, dusty and harsh environment in the sun. They were shown grabbing cold cans of full-strength beer and quenching their thirst through rapid consumption of the beer. Such rapid consumption of alcohol in harsh hot conditions is potentially harmful to the health and safety of drinkers. Such images and dialogue place drinkers and potential drinkers at significant risk of alcohol-related harm.

Responsible promotion and serving of alcohol is a major concern of government and the alcohol and hospitality industries in Australia. Self-regulation by the alcohol industry has resulted in improvements in serving and security practices in many licensed premises. These are reinforced through legislation and codes of practice developed and taken seriously by the industry. It is the irresponsible marketing of alcohol and the depiction of poor drinking behaviours which need to be stopped by the community.

Alcohol and violence

The relationship between intoxication and violence is complex and we need to be cautious about offering simple answers to complex issues in this regard. As a community we have difficulty in understanding and responding effectively to alcohol-related violence. Intoxication is the combination of the psycho-physical depressant effects of alcohol on the central nervous system; its manifestation is influenced by the intentions, attitudes and behaviours which the drinker brings to the situation.

Almost one in ten Australians suffer alcohol-related physical assaults. Males are more likely than females to be victims of such assaults, although females are still at significant risk. More than one-third of all Australians have suffered an alcohol-related verbal assault and 15 per cent have suffered property loss or damage in alcohol-related incidents (NDS,1995).

ALCOHOL USE AND INDIGENOUS AUSTRALIANS

It is difficult to highlight the threats to indigenous health from excessive use of alcohol without inflaming already negative beliefs about indigenous people, including those who drink. As Saggers and Gray (1991) have cautioned:

> Excessive use of alcohol has a significant role in Aboriginal morbidity and mortality. Unfortunately, racist discussion about the harmful role of alcohol in Aboriginal communities has meant that many social scientists are naturally cautious about adding to the public debate.

Contrary to myths in the general community, only 62 per cent of indigenous Australian men drink alcohol compared with 80 per cent of non-indigenous Australian men (Commonwealth Department of Human Services and Health,

1994a). Even fewer indigenous women drink. However, of those indigenous men who do drink, many consume alcohol at more harmful levels than do other drinkers in the general population.

The underlying conditions and reasons for heavy drinking amongst indigenous men are complex, with differences existing amongst individuals, groups and communities. Saggers and Gray (1991) explain that:

> Aboriginal drinking patterns are similar to those in other groups of impoverished, dispossessed peoples throughout the world.

TOBACCO USE

Tobacco is still the number one killer of drug users. Tobacco-related illnesses tend to manifest as smokers enter their mature adult years, causing chronic illness, reduced capacity to function and, often, premature death. In 1995 more than 22 500 people died from drug-related problems:

- 80.4 per cent of drug deaths were associated with tobacco;
- 16.2 per cent were linked to alcohol; and
- 3.5 per cent were from the use of illicit substances (Single and Rohl, 1997).

Tobacco adversely affects the health of both men and women. In 1995 the majority of tobacco-related hospital separations were amongst men aged 35 years or more (Single and Rohl, 1997). While fewer men smoke today than did in previous generations, there are still more men than women smoking — 27 per cent of males compared with 22 per cent of females (Single and Rohl, 1997). However, there seems to be a positive trend of reduced smoking rates amongst men. In 1995, 50 per cent of males aged 14–19 years had never smoked compared with 43 per cent in 1993. The smoking patterns of 14–19-year-old males remained the same in 1995 as in 1993 with 19 per cent smoking, but there has been a reduction in the numbers of male smokers aged 20–54 years (Single and Rohl, 1997). There is now evidence that the age at which people first try smoking is increasing. These encouraging figures may be due to the incremental effects of

- increased public awareness of the risks of smoking to health,
- stronger occupational health laws regarding smoking and passive smoking, and
- stricter laws prohibiting advertising of tobacco products.

ILLICIT DRUGS

Cannabis is the most widely used illegal drug in the Australian community, used by some 31 per cent of the population. It is consumed about six times more often than other illicit drugs such as heroin, amphetamines, ecstasy or

LSD (NDS, 1995). In 1995, 28 per cent of 14–19-year olds had used cannabis, with a decrease in use after the age of 34 years to around 5 per cent of 35–54-year olds (NDS, 1995). About 40 per cent of cannabis users use the drug occasionally and about a third on a weekly basis. More males than females have used or are currently using cannabis. This is an issue that needs to be addressed if men's health is to be improved.

Because cannabis is usually smoked, frequent or chronic use can lead to a real risk of lung and throat damage (Commonwealth Department of Human Services and Health, 1994b). This is particularly so if tobacco is mixed with cannabis and smoked. The combined use of tobacco, alcohol and cannabis can have adverse short-term and long-term effects. For example, using more than one depressant can cause:

- unpredictable and gross intoxication,
- impaired ability to manage the environment and
- other unwanted effects.

There are also risks of longer-term medical problems associated with combined use of tobacco, cannabis and alcohol, such as coronary heart disease, neck and throat cancer, lung disease and psychosocial problems (NDS,1995).

Cannabis also places the user at risk of accident due to an altered ability to perceive the environment. This affects driving and other activities requiring accuracy in decision-making, fine motor skills, and eye–hand coordination.

The use of illicit substances such as heroin, amphetamines and ecstasy is less common in the general adult population. The majority of users of ecstasy, amphetamines and hallucinogenics are 20–29 years old (Single and Rohl, 1997; NDS, 1995).

There appears to have been no increase in the use of heroin and cocaine between 1985 and 1995 (Single and Rohl, 1997). The rate of consumption of cannabis, amphetamines and ecstasy amongst young men has increased only slightly since 1985.

However, the human and material costs of illicit drug use are significant, despite these drugs being used by fewer people than those using alcohol and tobacco. In Australia in 1995 it is estimated that 778 young people died as a result of illicit drug use. Of these deaths four times more men than women died. More males than females use illicit drugs, placing significant numbers of men at risk of health, legal and social problems.

UNDERSTANDING DRUG-RELATED PROBLEMS

Males consume more alcohol more frequently than females, people who are divorced or never married are less likely to be abstinent than those who are in stable partnerships, and people who are unemployed are more likely to be abstinent of alcohol. However, people who drink and are poorly educated or unemployed are more likely to drink at hazardous/harmful levels when they drink, compared with the general population. Realising that there are connections between life situations and alcohol/drug use makes health workers more effective in understanding why people do or do not drink/use drugs, their patterns of consumption and what influences safe or unsafe use.

Improving men's health requires special attention to reaching the men who are in desperate need of help. Strategies such as the formation of men's groups need to be expanded to reach more men. Through recent research such as the National Drug Strategies from 1993 to 1997 the drug and alcohol field has developed a greater understanding of prevention and responses to drug-use problems in Australia. It is now known that all health workers (not just specialist drug and alcohol workers) need to understand, support, and provide education, assessment, interventions and referral for their clients regarding alcohol and drug use matters.

Many people reduce, alter or cease their alcohol or drug use themselves with little or no help from professionals or associates. This may be in response to an emotional or work problem, an accident or a change in role.

A major theme in all alcohol and drug work is that of providing a range of effective strategies to suit the current needs of a client. For example, there is little point in trying to influence young binge drinkers to be abstinent for the rest of their lives or a person experiencing severe dependence to have a social drink once a week with their drinking partners. There is also little sense in trying to convince someone who is in a family crisis to start a long-term therapy program when they do not even know where they are going to be living the next day.

Sensitivity of health workers can play an important role in responding to men's expressed needs. When workers apply a flexible approach to addressing alcohol and drug concerns, clients can be assisted in trusting themselves to make change in a supportive environment with the help of the worker. Clients can then develop their motivation, skills and energies to reclaim their balance and improve their wellbeing along the way.

BRIEF INTERVENTION

Brief intervention provides users with clear information about alcohol or drug use, advice about their own current use and any links to or likely harmful consequences of their use. Information can be provided through:

- written material,
- telephone advice or counselling,
- 'pen pal' correspondence with a health professional,

- self-help manuals or
- face-to-face discussions on issues.

As with many health concerns which people experience, brief intervention is valuable in assisting the person to identify their own issues, strategies, resources and solutions. Brief intervention has been shown to be very effective for people who are occasional to excessive drinkers or drug users (Mattick et al., 1993). Men who are not likely to benefit are those who are experiencing complex life issues and alcohol/drug dependency.

Examples of brief interventions are:

- a ten-minute education and discussion session on safe drinking with a patient in hospital,
- a short series of half-hour counselling sessions or
- provision of a once-off program using a video and discussion group amongst peers.

Brief interventions are opportunistic, can be applied wherever the client is and can occur in any health or community setting — hospitals, GPs' rooms, community nursing services, the home, culturally based services, community houses or church halls.

HARM REDUCTION

The basis of quality health care is to 'do no harm'. Where alcohol or drug use exists there is always the potential for risk of harm to individuals and the community. The principles and practices of harm reduction within public health and personal health care delivery are critical. Harm reduction encourages us to focus not only on obvious problems, such as addiction, but on the spectrum of alcohol and drug-use problems which may or do exist.

For people who inject drugs, the provision of clean injecting equipment through needle exchanges, education on safe injecting practices and overdose prevention packages minimise the risk of accidental overdose and the spread of blood-borne infections such as HIV and hepatitis amongst associates and the wider community. Access for alcohol and other drug users to social and health care support through GPs, local hospitals and community services is also effective in reducing harm.

Harm reduction is not exclusive to illicit drugs or alcohol use. There are now a range of resources available for smokers wishing to give up or reduce their smoking, including public information and education, self-help resources and counselling. Nicotine gum and patches can be prescribed to help overcome the addiction.

SERVICES

Referral and self-presentation to drug, alcohol and other relevant services are available in all states of Australia. Many services are free and provided by the public health system. Most people, however, do not require specialist services so local GPs, community nurses, general hospitals, community health centres and other health and social services are well able to assist in identifying and addressing alcohol or drug issues impacting on people's health and social lives. Self-help groups, anger management groups, general counselling, grief counselling, psychology and related services can all be helpful avenues for men experiencing alcohol and drug problems.

References

Collins D and Lapsley H (1996): *The social costs of drug abuse in Australia in 1988 and 1992.* Canberra: Australian Government Publishing Service.

Commonwealth Department of Human Services and Health (1994a): *National Drug Strategy Household Survey. Urban Aboriginal and Torres Strait Islander Peoples Supplement, 1994.* Canberra: Australian Government Publishing Service.

Commonwealth Department of Human Services and Health (1994b): *Handbook for Medical Practitioners and other Health Care Workers on Alcohol and Other Drug Problems.* Canberra: Australian Government Publishing Service

English D, Holman CD, Milne E and Winter M (1995): *The Quantification of Drug Caused Morbidity and Mortality in Australia.* Canberra: Commonwealth Department of Human Services and Health and Australian Government Publishing Service.

Fuchs C, Meir SJ, Colditz G, Giovannucci E, Manson JE, Kawachiet I, Hunter DJ, Hankinson SE, Hennekens CH, Rosner B, Speizer FE and Willett WC (1995): Alcohol consumption and mortality among women. *The New England Journal of Medicine* 332 19 May 11: 1245–1250.

Hall (1996): Head Space. *Centre Lines,* A quarterly newsletter from the National Centres for Drug and Alcohol Research, Sydney. Issue no. 29, September.

Mattick R, Baillie A, Grenyer B, Hall W, Jarvis T and Webster P (1993): An outline for the management of alcohol problems. Quality Assurance in the Treatment of Drug Dependence Project. National Drug Strategy. Canberra: Australian Government Publishing Service.

National Drug Strategy (NDS) (1994): *Statistics on Drug Abuse in Australia 1994.* Canberra: Department of Human Services and Health and Australian Government Publishing Service.

National Drug Strategy (NDS) (1995): *National Drug Strategy Household Survey. Survey Report 1995.* Canberra: Commonwealth Department of Health and Family Services and Australian Government Publishing Service.

Pols R and Hawks D (1992): *Is There a Safe Level of Daily Consumption of Alcohol for Men and Women?* Canberra: National Health and Medical Research Council and Australian Government Publishing Service.

Saggers S and Gray D (1991): *Aboriginal Health and Society. The Traditional and Contemporary Aboriginal Struggle for Better Health.* Australia: Allen and Unwin.

Single E and Rohl T (1997): *The National Drug Strategy: Mapping the Future. An Evaluation of the National Drug Strategy 1993–1997.* A report commissioned by the Ministerial Council on Drug Strategy, Commonwealth of Australia. Australia. Canberra: Australian Government Publishing Service.

Suggested reading

Brady M (1994): Drug and Alcohol Use among Aboriginal People. In: Reid and Trompf (eds) *The Health of Aboriginal Australia.* Australia: Harcourt Brace.

Committee for the Ministerial Council on Drug Strategy, Commonwealth of Australia (1993): *National Drug Strategy 1993. National Drug Strategic Plan 1993–9.* Canberra: Australian Government Publishing Service.

Cudmore M (1988): *History of the South Australian Brewing Company Limited 1888–1988.* South Australia: South Australian Brewing Company Ltd.

Gossop M (1996): *Living with Drugs* (4th edn). United Kingdom: Arena.

Keys and Young (1994): The incidence and prevalence of alcohol use and violence in the Australian community, Report 1 in a series of reports prepared for the National Symposium on Alcohol Misuse and Violence, Commonwealth of Australia. Canberra: Australian Government Printing Service.

Matthee R (1996): Exotic Substances: The Introduction and Global Spread of Tobacco, Coffee, Cocoa, Tea and Distilled Liquor, Sixteenth to Eighteenth Centuries. In Porter and Teich (eds): *Drugs and Narcotics in History.* United Kingdom: Cambridge University Press.

Pinger R, Payne W, Hahn D and Hahn E (eds) (1995): *Issues for Today: Drugs* (2nd edn). St Louis: Mosby.

Thorley A (1980): Medical responses to problem drinking. *Medicine* (3rd series) 35.

White J (1991): *Drug Dependence.* New Jersey: Prentice-Hall, Inc.

Zinberg N (1984): *Drug, Set, and Setting.* New Haven: Yale University Press.

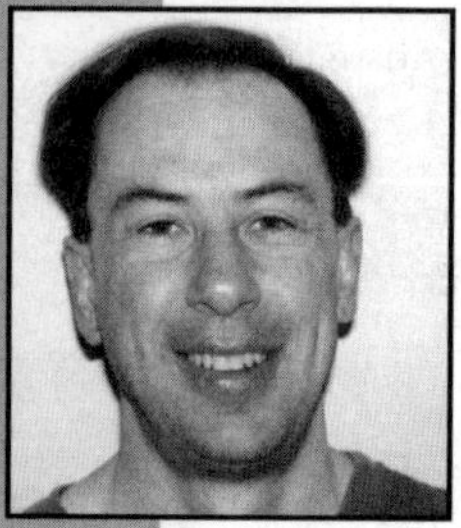

JAMES MABBUTT

Diploma of Science (Nursing), Bachelor of Nursing
Clinical Nurse Consultant, South West Sydney Community Health Area Drug and Alcohol Service

Of himself and this chapter, James said the following:
I am Sydney born and bred. I took up nursing when I was 23, which I feel was an advantage. I've enjoyed the opportunity to travel, live and work overseas. I have specialised in drug and alcohol work which first introduced me to men's health via a 'men's group' at a detoxification centre. I've also experienced the challenge of attending men's festivals and a weekly men's group and have personally gained a great deal from the support of the men involved. I am studying part-time for a master's degree in public health and searching continually for the place where men's health can fit into the health system. My interests include sleeping, eating, watching cricket and other more noble pursuits. I am married and living in the southern parts of Sydney.

This chapter is dedicated to my father, Geoff, who died suddenly in 1990, and to my grandfather, Frank, who was told to 'go home and be a man'. He did, and was dead a week later. It's time to challenge the way boys and men should be.

Chapter 6

The nurse's role in implementing men's health promotion programs in the Australian community

'work, consume, be silent, die'
— The wall, North Cronulla Beach, Sydney, 1980s

INTRODUCTION

Public health and primary health care are approaches to improving and promoting health in the Australian community. Public health targets the prevention of illnesses in men in the general population rather than in specific groups. Primary health care seeks to provide prevention and treatment to individuals and groups in local communities. Although at the surface level these approaches appear separate from each other, they work closely together and their programs can overlap.

This chapter will focus on primary health care and the benefits it brings to the Australian community and particularly to men within that community. The chapter will show that, guided by the health promotion principles outlined in the Ottawa Charter (World Health Organization, 1986), nurses can successfully implement and contribute to men's health promotion programs in their local community.

Although most nurses are employed in hospitals, the dividing line between hospitals and community-based services is becoming less defined. Local, community-based care (primary health care) continues to grow, with a strong influence on health promotion and illness prevention. Nurses have an important role in health promotion and, in many instances, nurses have a primary care role in which their level of independent practice is likely to increase (NHMRC, 1991:11). The role of a nurse involved in health promotion to reduce the risks of heart disease is very different from that of a nurse nursing men in a coronary care unit after they have had a myocardial infarct.

There needs to be a change in practice and in strategies that target men and involve them in improving their health.

As there is an increasing expectation that people will take control of their own health, the involvement of nurses in promoting self-determination can benefit men as a group and the community as a whole. Health promotion programs for men need to be delivered in a way that will engage men and empower them to take control of their own health needs, as individuals or as communities.

PUBLIC HEALTH

There are reasons why diseases occur in populations and the reasons are no longer seen as magical or the will of God. Public health investigations or population-based studies provide information on the prevalence and incidence of disease. The cause of illness can often be attributed to the behaviour of individuals, for example, smoking, harmful consumption of alcohol, dangerous driving and unsafe sexual practices. Illness in populations can generally be influenced by the social class of the person, their employment status, where they live and their environment. Diseases are not distributed by chance.

Three assumptions of public health are:

- diseases do not occur by chance;
- individual behaviours contribute to illness, disability and death; and
- diseases are not randomly distributed in populations (Baume, 1996:25).

Public health strategies are developed and advice is given to individuals to reduce the risk of disease. The national campaign in Australia against skin cancer, including the Anti-Cancer Council's strategy of 'Slip, Slop, Slap', is a recent example of the public health approach.

In terms of health equity, public health is concerned about identifying the disadvantage of groups within the population. Australian men have distinct health care problems but until recently they have been considered the norm. Consequently, few proactive measures have been used to reduce the relatively high mortality, morbidity and injury rates of men (Lawson, 1991:202). Subgroups of men — those with low socioeconomic status and Aboriginal and Torres Strait Islander men — have even higher levels of mortality and morbidity. The poor health status of disadvantaged groups within the male population can have a huge impact on the cost of health care in the community, and wider consequences of alienation within society.

Prevention of disease has been classified as

- primary — preventing disease before it occurs, and
- secondary, which relates to early intervention.

Two good examples of population-based secondary prevention opportunities for women have been cervical and breast cancer screening (Palmer and Short, 1994). However, opportunities to screen men for testicular cancer and prostate cancer have not been forthcoming as debate continues with respect to the effectiveness of screening in terms of changing the course of the disease (Palmer and Short, 1994).

PRIMARY HEALTH CARE

Primary health care involves providing health services at the first point of contact, with the attempt to meet health problems as soon as they arise. The intervention should be comprehensive, involving health practitioners working with nongovernment organisations and, especially, the community itself. To achieve self-reliance the community and individuals within it need to be involved in the planning, organisation and management of primary health care (World Health Organization, 1978). Nurses, as the largest health professional group, have an important role to play in primary health care provision.

Primary health care value in health service provision has been seen as an approach which balances prevention with treatment. Primary health care does involve the treatment of disease and disability but it also has a major emphasis on prevention of disease. The curative approach, which advocates treatment of health problems as they arise, overwhelms prevention in Australia. For example, in 1989–90 only 4.4 per cent of the health budget was spent on prevention (Wass, 1994). The disadvantage of the predominant treatment-focused health services is that long-term positive health outcomes of a population are decreased, and treating diseases caused by behavioural choices by people (e.g. heart disease, cancer and diabetes) may be more difficult and expensive than preventive measures (Palmer and Short, 1994).

HEALTH PROMOTION AND THE OTTAWA CHARTER

The Ottawa Charter was the result of the first International Conference on Health promotion held in Ottawa, Canada, in 1986 (World Health Organization, 1986). Health promotion practice was outlined in five areas of the Ottawa Charter:

- build healthy policy;
- create supportive environments;
- strengthen community action;
- develop personal skills; and
- reorientate health services.

Following the Second International Conference on Health Promotion, held in Adelaide in 1988, Australia embraced health promotion on the principles of the

Ottawa Charter (O'Connor and Parker, 1995). However, in Australian society, due to social and political issues, there has been a difficulty fitting men's health promotion programs into the Ottawa Charter model. But the Ottawa Charter is a model that should work with men because it encourages men to take control over their health.

NURSES' ROLE IN MEN'S HEALTH PROMOTION

Health promotion underpins the principles of primary health care and the literature calls for nurses to take up health promotion practice (Lindsey and Hartrick, 1996; Skinner, 1995; Wass, 1994; Wilson-Barnett and Macleod Clark, 1993).

The need for the promotion of health by nurses was recognised by Florence Nightingale who said

> Both kinds of nursing are to put us in the best possible conditions for Nature to restore or preserve health, to prevent or to cure disease and injury. (Wilson-Barnett and Macleod Clark, 1993:257)

Nursing practice remains based predominantly on the 'sick model' (Wilson-Barnett and Macleod Clark, 1993:257) whereas the practice of health promotion encourages involvement and cooperation between clients and professionals (Pike and Forster, 1995). Beaumont (1988:7) called for nurses to practice health promotion in an attempt to change social structure and build healthy public policy. In a study by James et al. (1990) the authors found that the role of health promotion was an important practice for nurses as key health professionals, especially in isolated areas. Nurses are 70 per cent of the paid health workforce so their potential impact in adopting health promotion cannot be overemphasised (Wass, 1994:13). These changes in practice need to be embraced by nurses at the very core of their practice.

Since the 1980s there has been a recognition by community groups and workers that men as a group have specific needs which require health promotion projects and from the very beginning, nurses have been involved. At a conference on men's health in Melbourne in November 1993, nurses were described as being at the forefront of this recognition (Fletcher, 1993, 1995). The Australian Government, in 1995, recognised the need by auspicing a National Men's Health Conference and a subsequent Draft National Health Policy (Commonwealth Department of Human Services and Health, 1996). Prior to this South Australia and Tasmania had strategically planned for men's health (Wadham, Bentley and Booth; Harris and Curran, 1996). In other parts of Australia there had been regional or local planning of health promotion programs for men, generally isolated from other projects.

Fareed (1994) and Williamson (1995) described the need for nurses to promote the health of men by education, advice, support and in partnerships with other workers who already have contact with groups of men. There are many examples of nurses being involved in men's health promotion projects, including 'stress management; testicular self-examination; occupational health; Men's Health Nurse Practitioner and Well Man Clinics' (Fletcher 1993:4).

HOW CAN NURSES IMPLEMENT MEN'S HEALTH PROMOTION PROGRAMS IN AUSTRALIA?

There are various types of health promotion programs that have targeted men in Australia. Traditionally health education programs have been used in health promotion to influence a change in the individual's behaviour and some have been designed to engage men and 'develop personal skills' as identified in the Ottawa Charter. Other health promotion initiatives have addressed the call of the Ottawa Charter to 'create supportive environments' and 'strengthen community action'. These locally based programs, working within the primary health care concept, attempt to give control of health issues to local communities so that they can be focused on the particular needs of the communities.

Some key issues are important when planning health promotion programs for men. These are considered below.

1. Advertising the program

Advertising is the key to ensuring attention from men in local communities and attendance at health education programs. Various forms of media should be used.(Donaldson, 1996; Williams and Were, 1993). Using the local newspapers, which are read by many partners of men, is one way of the information reaching men through someone else. Mabbutt and Graff (1995) found a significant difference in attendance in a health education program, based upon the amount of information in newspaper advertisements. Advertisements that gave information about why men should attend the program and what benefits it could give them were the most successful. In a city environment the distribution of fliers with limited information was not successful. In a rural community the use of fliers can have a more positive impact. Word of mouth is an important form of advertising.

It is important to advertise in the media used by the men being targeted. For example, safe sex messages targeting the gay community in Sydney during the initial spread of HIV and AIDS were and continue to be advertised in the gay media, not the general media. 'Quit smoking' messages for men from the Vietnamese community in southwest Sydney were and continue to be advertised in the Vietnamese media. There was even a billboard written in Vietnamese used in a local area.

To target the 'average man', that, is one unfamiliar with men's health education programs, it is important to mention such problems as heart disease, cancer or stress and to offer potential solutions to 'fix these problems' through attending the program. 'Fix-the-problem' advertising is effective if the men or their wives, partners or lovers relate to the topics that are promoted. This approach connects with lay people as it promotes the program on safe ground. Advertising 'discussion groups' on men's issues will not gain access to the 'average man' but he will attend a stress management program or a men's health evening. Advertising to the group of men who are targeted by the program is important, as is selling the program as a local initiative (Donaldson, 1996; Williams and Were, 1993).

2. Using appropriate language

Men relate well to language that means something to them; using language that women relate to may alienate men.

In Australia, a prime example was conducted in Alice Springs. Middle-aged men were targeted by promoting a health education program as a 'chassis check'. Men related well to the need for regular car services, which connected the program to their own health needs. The program was a great success because it used 'male-friendly language' and well-known local leaders. Donaldson (1996:262) encouraged the use of language that local people could understand. When men feel safe or in a 'comfort zone', barriers are removed and the opportunity arises for men to ask questions and take risks in the presence of other men. Men talk about their feelings in front of other men in safe environments (Myors and Mabbutt, 1997).

3. Giving control

It is important that, after the initial stages of a health education program, men are given some control and responsibility, as this leads to ownership of the issues and enhances involvement. Mabbutt and Graff (1995) found this in a health education program in which participants developed personal skills and confidence to become leaders. In a community-based health promotion program (Millan, 1996) control was given to the men targeted by using focus groups and then involving the men in decisions on the program activities. This helped encourage their participation and ownership of the project.

4. Men-only programs

Men discuss issues with other men that they would not discuss in the presence of women. In men-only health education programs there is a different interaction from that in a combined male and female group. In parenting education programs, men were demonstrated to benefit from separate gender groups because they could discuss issues relating to the emotional side of the transition to fatherhood (Myors and Mabbutt, 1997; Barclay et al., 1996; Schmied et al., 1994). Allen and Whatley (1986) claim that male nurses, as men, may also gain personal benefits from the men's health movement. Male nurses can help with the reorientation of health services toward more health promotion programs for men. In some areas where there are no male health workers to run programs, female leaders have taken on the role and initiated programs in a very competent way, thus continuing the drive for male-specific health promotion programs.

5. Cost of the program

Health education programs that target men from health disadvantaged groups, for example, Aboriginal and Torres Strait Islanders and groups of low socioeconomic status, have charged little or nothing in the way of fees but have still failed to attract any significant numbers of participants. The cost of the program is, therefore, excluded as a reason why men might not attend. Low-cost programs can play an important role in delivering health information and education for these groups. A program that charges fees to cover expenses is a reasonable guideline when alternative funding is not available.

There is also a body of thought that suggests a need to charge a substantial amount of money, otherwise men may feel that the program is not professional or worthwhile. This assumption may have a basis of truth in the general population but is usually reserved for personal development programs. It disadvantages men of low socioeconomic status.

Health education programs

There are some good guidelines for planning and delivering health education to men in Australia, for example, *Men's Health Manual, A Step-by-step Guide for Establishing a Men's Health Program* (Williams and Were, 1993) and *The Men and Stress Manual* (Mabbutt and Graff, 1995).

This following process, described by Williams and Were, is a guide to implementing a men's health education program in a local community:

1. Assess the needs (questionnaire)
2. Develop the course
3. Promote the course
4. Interview applicants to assess their suitability
5. Implement the course
6. Evaluate

The examples that follow demonstrate the use of this model to implement men's health education programs. Each example outlines a different program. The first, the Men and Stress Program, describes a men's health program held in a small-group setting, by health professionals, in a city environment. The second program, A Men's Night Out, outlines a locally run health information program conducted in rural Victoria and delivered to a large group of men.

Men and Stress Program

In 1990 James Mabbutt and Bruce Graff adapted a program previously conducted by Hunt and Hickey (1989). The adaptation was to conduct a structured stress management program for the first three sessions then negotiate with the men to choose the content of the next three sessions. The adaptation was designed to stimulate the facilitators to develop new teaching material, and to empower the men to make choices regarding their personal needs in relation to stress in their lives (Mabbutt and Graff, 1995).

The program was advertised in the local paper. In most cases the men's wives/partners made the bookings. The program was facilitated by male health professionals. It was conducted in a number of community health centres in the area.

The program was evaluated by the participants at the end of each session and at the end of the course. Early in the course, participants were asked to state their objectives in attending. Evaluation at the end of the program involved review of these objectives. The evaluations demonstrated that the men found the program worthwhile and enlightening. The program had the advantage of engaging the general male population in a health promotion course which was advertised as 'fixing the problem'. This type of program could be used in many different settings.

A Men's Night Out

In 1993, Anne Donaldson, a community nurse from country Victoria, felt there was a need to provide a venue for men to discover health-related issues so she initiated, planned and presented a program called A Men's Night Out (Donaldson, 1995).

The program took the form of a cabaret with speakers presenting between the courses of an evening meal. The program was aimed at preventive health by providing a comfortable environment for men to meet and learn about stress, heart disease and prostate problems. The program also encouraged men to support each other in a rural setting in ways not previously explored. The first program was delivered to 160 men in the local area. Support was given by community groups and local businesses. Subsequently the program was delivered in other areas of Victoria, with similar large attendances.

Advertising the program was considered a key point in targeting rural men. The program was accessible only to men as past attempts to develop a men's health program had resulted in wives and partners attending instead, which did not allow men to ask questions that concerned them. Speakers were encouraged to use anecdotes with which the men were able to identify. Evaluations completed at the end of each program were very positive and demonstrated that the barriers of nonattendance at health promotion programs for men had been broken in rural communities. The program has since been implemented in different parts of Victoria and beyond, sponsored and run by local Lions groups, which provides an excellent example of the development of community responsibility. The success of the first A Men's Night Out stimulated the local community health service to conduct further men's health programs.

These two examples represent the Ottawa Charter in action in Australia. They demonstrate how to 'develop personal skills' in small or larger group settings and A Men's Night Out also incorporated the ability to 'strengthen community action' when local organisations adopted the program and ran it themselves with the assistance of speakers from health services. Both programs challenged the existing health services by providing programs for men specifically in a health promotion framework.

The Health is Gold project

In 1993 a project commenced in the South Western Sydney Area Health Service to address the problem that Vietnamese men had much higher rates of smoking than the general community (Rissel and Russel, 1992). 'The goal of the project was to reduce the prevalence of smoking among Vietnamese men' in the area (Mitchell et al., 1995). The project attempted to increase awareness of the health risks of smoking and increase the men's readiness and attempts to quit.

This project is an example of a men's health promotion project using intersectoral collaboration between an ethnic community in Australia and a health service. A full-time, male health promotion worker, Khoa Nguyen, was employed for the project. The initial working party comprised members from the area drug and alcohol and health promotion units, a local community health service, the Drug and Alcohol Multi Cultural Education Centre (DAMEC) and the NSW Quit Campaign (Nguyen, 1996). Nurses were involved in the working party to implement the project. This core working group involved the Vietnamese community in the project in all levels of implementation, ongoing planning and intervention. Representatives of Vietnamese organisations were involved in the project, including the Vietnamese Health Professionals Association of NSW and Vietnamese community workers from government and nongovernment organisations.

The project used culturally targeted posters and ethnic media in an attempt to offer community and/or family support for Vietnamese males to cease smoking. The Vietnamese community did not identify tobacco as a drug so an objective of the program was to change this attitude. It was hoped that a combination of awareness and change in attitude would lead to an increase in attempts to cease smoking. Pre and post surveys of these objectives were conducted. They revealed a decrease in the number of male smokers and an increase in attempts to cease smoking.

The Health is Gold Project demonstrated the ability within a defined community to 'create a supportive environment' for men to stop smoking or attempt to quit. The Vietnamese community supported the project and there was a 'strengthening of community action' through a process of an intersectoral approach, consultation with the community and education. The success of the program influenced other health services to implement similar projects recognising the need to 'reorientate health services' towards such health promotion projects. General practitioners were also trained to deliver culturally appropriate 'quit smoking' interventions, thus further reorientating health training needs in this area.

Gay Men Fighting AIDS

Greg Millan, a health promotion officer, commenced in the Gay Men Fighting AIDS project in 1994. The project sought to:

> minimise the transmission of HIV, optimise the health quality of people living with HIV/AIDS and address other related gay men's health issues (Millan, 1995, 1996).

The project was conducted by the Central Sydney Area Health Service which had high numbers of gay and lesbian residents; for example, gay and lesbian people in one suburb accounted for 25 per cent of the population. Lack of services or support groups for gay men was identified as a problem in the area. The project consulted the gay community through community meetings and monthly newsletters which encouraged the community to participate in various activities to meet the objectives.

It is believed that one reason for the success of the project was that it targeted gay men only. The project encouraged gay men to take action to improve their health and the health of the community. The consultations led to the decision that all gay men should be included in the project regardless of their HIV status. The response from the gay community was positive. Gay men welcomed the opportunity to take control of the process, identifying their needs and how best to address them.

The Gay Men Fighting AIDS project consultation process continues to engage the gay community, which has responded to the opportunity to take control over issues involving their health. Community participation in the project demonstrates the success of connecting with a community and the benefits of ownership by men who share similar health needs. Although nurses were not involved in the management of the project they contributed by conducting education sessions, by themselves being part of the consultation process and by creating supportive environments in their own communities to assist the gay community.

Evaluation issues

In Australia, process evaluation of men's health programs has been an accepted practice. Process evaluation often uses questionnaires, surveys and other measures before and/or after the program to measure its effect. In health education programs each session of the program may be evaluated which is a useful method to develop and refine programs. In a community-wide program pre and post surveys conducted in the community will give an indication as to the success of the program.

Few impact and outcome evaluation studies have been completed on men's health promotion programs in Australia. Evaluation that demonstrates health outcome benefits for the participants is difficult to implement with short-term funding and limited resources. Impact and outcome evaluation which demonstrates positive benefits for participants has the potential to increase funding for men's health initiatives, and should be attempted as a priority. There is also a need to 'write up' programs for publication in conference proceedings or referred journals.

MEN'S HEALTH PROMOTION PROGRAMS FOR THE FUTURE

Interest is increasing in men's health promotion programs in Australia. Many public health practitioners, however, claim there is no benefit in targeting men. This is despite the fact that men have benefited from population-based programs in the past, for example, heart disease. It is argued that screening men specifically for risk factors associated with heart disease (Leeder and Orr 1996:76) and prostate screening (Lange 1995:viii) has no cost benefits.

The slow shift of practice is a change of mind from focusing on the individual to supporting the community to change itself. It is too early to prove that these programs have improved the long-term health outcomes for men. The task of demonstrating the benefits of these programs is further complicated by other Australia-wide programs or local health promotion programs being conducted at the same time (National Health Strategy, 1993:103). However, from a qualitative and process evaluation perspective, there is evidence to demonstrate that local men's health promotion programs have been effective.

As men's health promotion programs become more accepted in their own right, programs will be available to target groups of men who have a poor health status. Nurses, particularly in the community, are well positioned to take up the challenge of providing health promotion programs for men. The examples described in this chapter show a shift from the predominantly small-group health education programs to local community programs that target men from different groups. Although nurses did not initiate all these examples they supported the programs and have skills in their own right to develop new and innovative programs in the future. The biggest challenge is to find fresh ways to gain access to men who do not benefit from current programs and for nurses to discover resources to conduct programs. Such information is often passed on by word of mouth. The rewards for nurses in this adventure are inspiring; the journey is difficult but wholly worthwhile

Acknowledgements

Thank you to my wife, Karen Myors, who encouraged me to put in an abstract and take the opportunity that I had been talking about for a while. She then rescued me from a great dark pit of despair and helped me change a bunch of words into something with meaning.

And thanks to these people and any others who have supported me in writing this chapter or, in the past, in men's health work: Adrian Bauman, Paula Cheng, Anne Donaldson, Bruce Graff, Jenny Grosvenor, Greg Millan, Julie Nolan, Cathy Richardson, Jan Ritchie, Wendy Wickes and the staff at Liverpool Hospital Library.

References

Allen D and Whatley M (1986): Nursing and men's health. *Nursing Clinics of North America* 21 1: 3–13.

Barclay L, Donovan J and Genovese A (1996): Men's experiences during their partner's first pregnancy: a grounded theory analysis. *Australian Journal of Advanced Nursing*: 13 3: 12–24.

Baume P (1996) In: Baume P and Bauman A (eds) *Public Health an Introduction.* Centre for Public Health, University of NSW: Eriador Press, p. 25.

Beaumont M (1988): Nurses — invisible in health promotion? Editorial. *Australian Journal of Advanced Nursing* May 17 17: 7.

Commonwealth Department of Human Services and Health (1996): *Draft Men's Health Policy.*

Commonwealth of Australia (1996): *Proceedings from the National Men's Health Conference, 10–11 August 1995.* Canberra: Australian Government Publishing Service.

Darling Downs Region Health Promotion Unit (1995): Proceedings from the Men's Health Conference, 'Promoting the cause'. September.

Donaldson A (1996): *'A Men's Night Out'.* National Men's Health Conference. Canberra: Australian Government Publishing Service, pp. 260–3.

Fareed A (1994): Equal rights for men. *Nursing Times* 90 5: 26–9.

Fletcher R (1993): Men's Health Promotion: A Leading Role for Nurses. *Men's Health, the Forgotten Issue.* Melbourne: Ausmed Publications.

Fletcher R (1994): *Men's Health.* Australian Community Health Association, p.11.

Fletcher R (1995): *An Introduction to the New Men's Health.* University of Newcastle: Men's Health Project.

Harris E, Wise M, Hawe P, Finlay P and Nutbeam D (1995): *Working Together — Intersectoral Action for Health.* Canberra: Australian Government Publishing Service.

Harris T and Curran G (1996): *Men's Health Policy Development — Tasmania.* National Men's Health Conference. Canberra: Australian Government Publishing Service, pp. 220–2.

Hunt G and Hickey B (1989): *Men and Stress.* Proceedings from the Australian Community Health Association National Conference, 'Health promotion, the community health approach', Australian Community Health Association, pp. 184–6.

Jackson C (1993): Pitching the message at men. *Health Visitor* September 66 9: 327–8.

James R, Henrikson D, Steiner C and Golds M (1990): Case study: disease prevention — new roles for nurses in rural Australia. *Patient Education and Counselling* 16: 43–5.

Lange D (1995): Proceedings, Men's Health Conference, 'Promoting the cause'. Darling Downs Region Health Promotion Unit, September, p. viii.

Lawson J (1991): *Public Health Australia, An Introduction.* Sydney: McGraw-Hill, p. 202.

Leeder S and Orr N (1996): *Heart Disease and Men's Health.* National Men's Health Conference. Canberra: Australian Government Publishing Service, pp. 73–6.

Lindsey E and Hartrick G (1996): Health-promoting nursing practice: the demise of the nursing process? *Journal of Advanced Nursing* 23: 106–12.

Mabbutt J and Graff B (1995: *Men and Stress Program Manual,* St George Community Health Drug and Alcohol Team, (2nd updated edn). Sydney: St George Hospital Drug and Alcohol Unit.

Millan G (1996): *Reclaiming Our Future, A Report on the Development of 'Gay Men Fighting Aids',* A Project of Central Sydney Area Health Service.

Millan G (1995): *Gay Men Fighting AIDS.* National Men's Health Conference. Canberra: Australian Government Publishing Service, pp. 251–4.

Mitchell J, Richardson C and Nguyen DK (1995): *Evaluation of a Vietnamese Anti-Smoking Project.* Conference Proceedings of the World Conference of the International Union for Health Promotion and Education, August.

Myors K and Mabbutt J (1997): *Gender Specific Groups: Is There a Need in Parent Education? TheExperiences of the Facilitators and the Couples.* 'The Truth, Virtue and Beauty of Midwifery', Australian College of Midwives 10th Biennial National Conference Proceedings, Melbourne, April.

National Health and Medical Research Council (1991): *The Role of the Nurse in Australia.* Canberra: Australian Government Publishing Service, p 11.

National Health Strategy (1993): *Pathways to Better Health,* Issues Paper No.7, March, Ch7, p.103.

Nguyen D (1996): Health is Gold, A Vietnamese Quit Smoking Program — Progress Report. South Western Sydney Area Health Service (unpublished).

O'Connor ML and Parker E (1995): *Health Promotion: Principles and Practice in the Australian Context.* St Leonards, New South Wales, Australia: Allen and Unwin.

Palmer GR and Short SD (1994): *Health Care and Public Policy,* 2nd edn. South Melbourne: Macmillan Education.

Pike S and Forster D (1995): *Health Promotion for All.* Churchill Livingstone.

Rissel C and Russel C (1992): *Heart disease risk factors in the Vietnamese community of south western Sydney.* Australian Journal of Public Health 17 1: 71–73.

Ritchie JE (1991): From health education to education for health in Australia: a historical perspective. *Health Promotion International*: 6 2: 157–63.

Schmied V, Wyllie A, Barclay L, Everitt L and Rogan F (1994): 'A sense of "readiness": women's reflections on their preparation for birth and parenting'. *'Families Our Future — Preconception to Parenthood', Proceedings of the Fourth Biennial Conference of the National Association of Childbirth Educators*, Canberra, September.

Skinner J in Pike S and Forster D (1995): *Health Promotion for All.* Churchill Livingstone.

St John W (1993): Primary health care: a clarification of the concept and the nursing role. *Contemporary Nurse*: 2 2: 73–8.

Wadham B, Bentley M and Booth A (1996): *Strategic Directions for Men's health: Therapy or Reform?* National Men's health Conference. Canberra: Australian Government Publishing Service, pp. 213–20.

Wass A (1994): *Promoting Health — The Primary Health Care Approach.* Sydney: W.B. Saunders/Baillere Tindall.

Williams P and Were T (1993): *Men's Health Manual A Step-by-step Guide for Establishing a Men's Health Program.* PO Box 572, Glenorchy, Tasmania.

Williamson P (1995): Their own worst enemy. *Nursing Times*: November 29, 91 48: 25–7.

Wilson-Barnett J and Macleod Clark J (1993): *Research in Health Promotion and Nursing* Great Britain: The Macmillan Press Ltd.

World Health Organization (1986): *Ottawa Charter for Health Promotion.* Ottawa, Canada: World Health Organisation.

World Health Organization (1986): *Intersectoral Action for Health.* Geneva: WHO.

World Health Organization (1978): *Primary Health Care.* International Conference on Primary Health Care, Alma Ata, USSR. Geneva and New York: WHO, UNICEF.

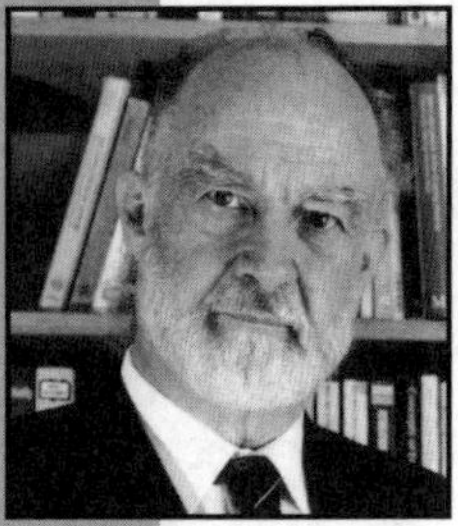

ELERY HAMILTON-SMITH

Professor and Honorary Research Fellow, Lincoln Gerontology Centre, La Trobe University, Melbourne, Australia

Elery Hamilton-Smith has more than 45 years' experience in social research and social planning, having worked at the community level, then as a social planning consultant across some 25 countries and, eventually, as a member of the Leisure Studies Department at Preston (later Phillip) Institute of Technology, which is now part of RMIT University in Melbourne. Elery has wide-ranging interests in social policy and social development, has been a visiting professor at many universities in North America and Europe and is currently a professor at the International Centre of Excellence at the University of Wageningen in the Netherlands. His long-standing interest in leisure services led to his involvement in a research program on improving the lot of people with a dementing illness. That research culminated in the development of the ELTOS (Enhanced Living Through Optimal Stimulus) theory and the book *Rethinking Dementia — an Australian approach* (of which he was joint Editor) with its companion kit *Teaching About Dementia*, both of which have sold widely in Australia and are now beginning to penetrate overseas. Elery describes himself as 'a sociologist by discipline, interested in almost everything, including social theory and research methods, parks and speleology'.

Chapter 7

ENHANCING MEN'S HEALTH

INTRODUCTION

At present in Australia, men are obviously much less healthy than women, in terms of both mortality and morbidity. Of course, gender comparisons are not all that useful, but they do demonstrate dramatically the nature of the men's health problem, and they do need consideration in the allocation of medical and other resources. Let me just make a few points about the current state of affairs :

- At birth, males have a life expectancy some 6 years less than females.
- Males have a higher incidence and higher death rate from virtually all illnesses (except breast cancer and ailments of the female reproductive system).
- Males have one of the highest suicide rates in the world and account for 80 per cent of all suicides in Australia.
- Males account for 95 per cent of the prison population.
- Males have some 95 per cent of workplace fatalities and permanent disabilities from workplace injuries.

At the same time, we must remember that some aspects of men's health are improving, and that most aspects of this improvement are due to social and cultural change: men spend much less time in smoke-filled bars drinking excessive amounts of beer; work conditions occasion less physical risk; nutrition is generally better. But, on the other hand, with the rise of economic rationalism and the associated managerialism, men are subject to immense increases in stress.

We also need to spend a minute on the strange anomaly that, while men at all ages have higher mortality rates than women, women appear to suffer a much higher morbidity level (Broom, 1989). Women, particularly with the social and cultural changes of the last 40 years, are more subject than men to external pressures of the kind which are likely to diminish trust in their own powers of discrimination, and in their own capacity for joy. This may generate wellness problems and constraints of a different kind from those suffered by men, and are not the business of this chapter. However, it needs be noted here, to make the point once again, that wellness has a whole range of gender-based dimensions.

Even more importantly, women have been socialised to admit and deal with fear, sorrow or other potentially negative emotions. They are not seen as 'weakies' if they go to a doctor; they are allowed to cry; they are allowed to admit to human frailty. So they report their ailments and become part of the morbidity statistics. Men pretend they are OK.

Similarly, women admit they find the balancing of work, childcare and spousecare demanding and potentially stressful — but they find ways of relieving and moderating that stress. As an indicative example, Bolger et al. (1989) found that women do not bring work stress home into the family situation; men do. This is further supported by British research reported at a Brisbane conference on stress which found that women's morbidity was strongly correlated with the nature of their spouse's occupation (*Age*, 11 March 1996). Not only are men badly impacted by stress; they inflict that stress upon others.

Overall, men are exposed to a wide range of stressors, many of them different from those of 15 years ago. Men are not prepared, by their socialisation or in any other way, to deal with these stressors. So, at an extreme, men suicide, or, on the other side of the coin, turn to violence or to workplace bullying (Rees, 1995). It can only be a matter of concern that young men are now dying in increasing numbers as a result of urban violence. At a less obvious level, stress impacts strongly upon the operation of the immune system, so it is not surprising that men's health is poor.

My approach to this topic is based in the fact that I am a sociologist, and have spent many years working in various areas, all concerned with the enhancement of lifestyle. Many stressors arise out of our lifestyle, so I have chosen to discuss four aspects of salutogenic (health-producing) behaviour which are certainly not the only ones that might be discussed, but are very directly relevant to lifestyle:

- personal and social relationships
- the extent to which we might or might not develop a consuming life-interest (or interests) in something
- the extent to which we might maintain an adequate level of physical activity
- maintenance of a positive mood, which sustains and at the same time, grows out of a coherent lifestyle.

PERSONAL AND SOCIAL RELATIONSHIPS

The importance of personal and social relationships has long been recognised in both common wisdom and cultural behaviour. All successful cultures provide various structural opportunities for the development of personal and social relationships, some of them more successfully than others. It is surely significant that the first-ever sociological monograph, Emile Durkheim's 1897 *Suicide*, found that the tragedy of suicide grew out of social relationships that lacked balance between individuality and social solidarity. As society moves increasingly towards the chaos of 'disorganised capitalism' (Offe, 1985) and more recently into economic rationalism as a typical 'putting-the-clock-back' response, current social theory is returning to address this issue once more. For instance, Benhabib (1992) talks of 'situating the self' and provides us with an exciting theoretical framework within which we might address the contemporary plight of the person.

But to address first the role of personal and social relationships in the genesis of wellness, we need to turn to the middle-range research which has taken place in the 95-year interval between Durkheim and Benhabib. A range of researchers have shown the extent to which the breakdown of relationships between individuals and their society is germane to problems of social disorder such as crime. But, some 25 years ago, Caplan (1974), Cassel (1976) and others commenced to examine psychosocial elements in the etiology of illness. They were able to argue a strong and probably causative relationship between illness and a breakdown in what they 'social support'. This served to commence a whole new generation of epidemiological studies which gave attention to the social environment; these have been comprehensively reviewed by House, Landis and Umberson (1988) and shown to have produced very convincing evidence indeed that a low score on 'social network' indices does have a strong impact upon mortality rates. Some of the studies that they reviewed also showed that a low score on 'social network' indices gave rise to higher rates of morbidity and slower recovery rates. Although current studies point to the need for further refinements in methodology and further testing of intervening variables (including gender), House et al. summarised their findings by arguing that the evidence was at least as powerful as that which led to the 1964 report by the US Surgeon-General that cigarette smoking was a major 'cause or risk factor for mortality and morbidity from a range of diseases'.

Just as further research on the impact of smoking has greatly strengthened the evidence, so new studies on social relationships are greatly strengthening the case for social relationships as a major force in wellness. Given this, together with the fact that Australia has one of the world's highest suicide rates amongst males, we now need to turn specifically to the evidence about male relationships.

Many relationship studies have demonstrated that the risk generated by poor relationships is much stronger in men than women (see the summary in House et al., 1998; also Nardi, 1992). They have also suggested variation between cultural groups (e.g. between rural and urban societies, or between various ethnic groups), but there is insufficient evidence yet to develop generalised statements at this level. Regrettably, while epidemiological studies have been able to identify the strength of the linkage between wellness and social relationships, they cannot help us understand the processes which make for good or bad relationships, nor those through which relationships actually enhance wellness. A further regrettable deficiency in the research is that a generation of researchers has assumed that the enhancement of wellness grows out of 'social support' (however defined), rather than seeking to elucidate the complex mix of processes that are involved.

The result is a massive body of work on social support (e.g. Sarason, Sarason and Pierce, 1990) which has led us little further forward. My personal view is that it has done little more than to show we need much more than a superficial, even trivialised, notion of social support to be of any value at all. Only a few researchers have yet departed from this social support model, and sought to elucidate the processes which actually take place. Rook (1990) has argued that companionship is more significant than support, and that such processes as the stimulation of arousal and positive affect, the shifting of attention away from mundane concerns or problems, the affirmation of self, distraction from undue self-scrutiny and the provision of companionship without the ambiguity of explicit social support are all important. Similarly in Australia, Gibson and Mugford (1986) have pointed to the role of confidants, the sense of acceptance, reassurance of one's own worth, and opportunities for joint participation. A further vital insight comes from Rawlins (1992) who demonstrated the inevitably dialectic nature of friendship. This certainly proved to be central to an investigation by a group of my own research students (in press), admittedly looking only at women's friendships and their linkage to wellness. Almost by definition, any study which neglects the dialectic element in friendship is guilty of oversimplification. These last studies certainly lead us to the sense that understanding the role of friendships in wellness must be rooted in a broadly based theory which can encompass both one's sense of self, and of how one relates to and finds meaning in wider society.

There are some very specific problems about relationships which face men. One of these is the cultural emphasis on sexuality in male personal relationships (Rawlins, 1992); two men who form a close personal friendship are suspected to be homosexuals, and despite some more enlightened attitudes, there is still widespread disapproval and marginalisation of male homosexuality (Miller, 1983); those who enjoy close cross-gender relationships are assumed to be sexual partners. In fact, this assumption is so pervasive that Wright (1989) sees the question of whether nonsexual cross-gender friendships even exist as central to any discussion of the topic.

There is also good evidence that men grow up in a cultural context which differs from that of women; Maccoby (1990) in the United States and Crawford et al. (1992) have drawn attention to the extent to which men and women are socialised to construct reality in quite different ways, and that as one result of this, men are likely to devalue intimacy in personal relationships, to repress any expression of emotion, and hence to avoid confronting any personal problems.

A third problem lies in aspects of contemporary cultural change. Male social relationships have traditionally been largely based in all-male groupings of sporting companions, drinking schools, workmate associations and the like. Even in this pattern, there were some problems; such groups often supported and reproduced cultural values, e.g. 'toughness', devaluation of women and the development of androcentric concepts of power (again at the expense of women) which are now rejected and which may well have been seriously detrimental to wellness. More importantly, these groups often consist of rivals rather than supporters (e.g. those rivalling one for promotion at work or success in team selection on the sports field) and so were people-who-must-be-reckoned-with more than friends in the full sense generally given to that word. As the work environment becomes more competitive, so it will probably be much less able to provide a satisfying network of friendships. Wellman (1992), in a Toronto-based study, argued that the communities of both men and women have increasingly become based in private and domestic spaces; that wives often maintain their partners' social networks and that men get a great deal of their emotional support from women, while women find almost all of their emotional support in relationships with other women. Wellman speculates that the definition of friendship seems to have narrowed to emotional support and companionship, and that at the same time, men's communities have shifted from public spaces to the private space of homes. All of this sounds very like the Australian experience, but it must be recognised, as with all cultural change, that these patterns are not distributed across the total population; they have affected the more affluent, upwardly mobile earlier and more deeply than the under-classes.

In summary, although one might wish for more research and knowledge, it is clear that friendship patterns are a very real determinant of wellness, that they generally have more impact upon men than on women, that they operate and are linked to wellness through a complex range of processes, and that there are a greater number of barriers in the way of men finding satisfactory personal relationships than there once were. It would seem then, that rather than producing further empirical research, it is important to develop a more robust theoretical framework about the idea of personal and social relationships so that the research which already exists can be grounded more adequately. I will return to this idea, but I turn now to the issue of life-interests.

LIFE-INTERESTS AND COMMITMENT

For some years, Robert Stebbins of Canada has been writing about what he calls 'serious leisure' (e.g. 1992). By this term, he means activities that involve the participant in a long-term commitment. He uses as examples the various ways in which people become amateurs or hobbyists, or work as long-term volunteers. I personally believe he has neglected the importance of community or political activism here, and there may well be other forms of commitment that might be included. Much more importantly, Lobo (1997) studied the outcomes of redundancy amongst middle-aged men: those who are made redundant at just the time when they would have expected to be at the most productive and successful stage of their career. Lobo found that one of the most important characteristics of those who adjust to and manage this experience with relative success is that they have some central life-interest other than their occupation, or in other words, 'serious leisure' as Stebbins would define it.

It is clear that this is not simply because these men have something 'to fill their time', even though that may in itself be important. Rather, such an interest feeds into the way in which we each define ourselves and the way in which others may perceive us. Lobo (1997) emphasises this by using the term 'leisure capital' to describe its value as a personal and social resource. It becomes part of our construction of self and of our place within society. So, when the world of work fails us by rejecting us, an alternative identity and social place remains intact. Lobo reported (and I have encountered similar examples) that some men turn their life interest into a new self-employed career, so that it may also serve an economic function.

As a lifetime amateur in various areas, I know personally how well my amateurism has served me in maintaining a healthy sense of self; in building an immense network of friendships; and even in enhancing my career. One of the issues which calls out for further thinking and research here is the extent to which some interests are structured to provide a greater range of developmental opportunities than others. Many competitive sports are structured so as to provide relatively few roles other than that of player or spectator; many of the now-commercialised opportunities for 'collecting' provide few opportunities for development and lifetime continuity; but others of the more traditional pursuits offer an almost endless number of specialised avenues. Studies of leisure specialisation (summarised in Hamilton-Smith, 1981) are amongst the few that give us any deeper understanding of how activities vary in their structural complexity, and hence, opportunity structure. An important benefit which accrues from most forms of serious leisure is the generation of networks of social relationships and friendships where common interest brings together otherwise diverse people, and provides one of the few opportunities in our kind of society for cross-generational friendships.

Both social relationships and expressed life-interests come together in most discussions about the nature of personal identity or sense of self, and in the building of self-esteem. Self develops out of what we do, and the way in which others perceive us, value us and relate to us.

PHYSICAL ACTIVITY AND WELLNESS

Ornstein and Sobel (1989), in their seminal book, *Healthy Pleasures* (which their publishers, for some strange reason, refuse to distribute in Australia) have a chapter titled, 'Why kill yourself to save your life?', in which they confront and challenge the fitness myth. One of the continuing problems of men's health (now invading the world of women) is the confused, uninformed thinking which sees fitness and wellness as synonymous. People are urged to pursue a fitness regime, ostensibly for the sake of their health, but probably more for the sake of the immense profits generated by the fitness industry. However, this confusion also invades a great deal of research; for instance, while Canada has conducted a national survey of wellness, Australia is still carrying out fitness surveys, and using the results of these to prescribe for wellness.

There is no question that physical activity is fundamental to wellness; the evidence is completely unequivocal. But there are significant problems with the fitness model — it leads to an immense number of injuries, often minor, but cumulatively serious; enjoyment is often neglected in exercise prescription and the targets set for individuals are often seen as excessive, and so compliance rates are poor; and the level of activity demanded is far in excess of the optimal level from a wellness perspective. The best health accrues to those who are only moderately active for some 30 minutes each day; greater exertion does not increase the health benefits, and often leads to damage. In fact, one of the major problems arising from the emphasis upon sport and exercise in Australia is the remarkable rate of accident and injury, which costs us in excess of one billion dollars per annum.

A further element hidden here is the whole question of the physical environment in which we might pursue any activity. There is now a significant accumulation of evidence that exposure to the natural environment lowers stress levels, and hence enhances wellness, in human beings (Ulrich, Dimberg and Driver, 1991). Human beings evolved within the natural environment, and at one time, physical activity would have been based in the active process of managing the interface with that environment. The resultant benefits to the organism would have been optimised. Today, with the industrialisation of sport and fitness, opportunities for exposure to the natural are seriously diminished. Walking through a park or doing one's own gardening are likely to do far more good to people than any number of hours spent in a gymnasium!

Again, the extent and nature of one's physical activity may be interrelated with one's other life-interests, and may serve to generate wider networks of social relationships and friendships.

KEEPING IN A GOOD MOOD

The Ornstein and Sobel book is based in the simple idea that experiences which are promoting of health and wellness, i.e. survival, will be pleasurable ones, simply because this ensures their continuation. This leads to their underlying assumption that 'the healthiest people seem to be pleasure-loving, pleasure-seeking, pleasure-creating individuals'. Pleasure is creative of wellness, but the definition of pleasure is not as easy as it sounds. We have been socialised to see a whole number of commercially provided entertainments as productive of pleasure (even if they are not) and many of us lose insight into the sources of our own happiness.

The idea of mood also goes hand-in-hand with the earlier discussion of commitment to a central life-interest. Csikszentmihalyi (1975, 1990), in his examination of autotelic behaviour, has shown how people can become totally involved in the experience of an activity to which they are committed, and in which the challenge or difficulty faced is matched by their own capacities. He used the term 'flow' to designate this state of enhancement of mood and pleasure. More recently, Csikszentmihalyi and Kleiber (1991) have discussed the issues in making this level of experience more universally available.

Returning to the'pleasure principle', the development of a positive, future-looking and essentially optimistic mood goes hand-in-hand with pleasure in life; it is another chicken-and-egg situation, where a positive mood state both grows out of and leads to a pleasurable lifestyle.

This brings me to look at one of the sets of theoretical ideas which point to a relatively satisfactory explanation of the way in which all the processes discussed here are linked to wellness, and the immense impact which they may have.

COHERENCE IN LIFE

It is now useful to turn to a broader and more robust concept, which is Antonovsky's (1979, 1987) concept of coherence. Antonovsky was perhaps most easily described as a health sociologist, but I am sure he would not have liked that term, as he was at pains to make the point that he was interested in wellness, and in his belief, that is a much broader and quite different idea. He was long concerned with the question of why and how some people remain well, even though exposed to risks and stressors that would cause others to become ill. In examining the various social mechanisms that maintain wellness, including those which I have discussed here, he came to the conclusion that the central factor in wellness is the development of a Sense of Coherence, which enables people to mobilise resistance to risks or stressors.

This is a remarkably comprehensive idea; it involves not only a robust sense of self, but an appreciation and understanding of the ways in which that self is rooted in culture. More specifically, it includes an understanding of our own situation which enables us to see events as explicable and more-or-less predictable, a sense of our own capacity to manage risks and stressors, and a sense that life is meaningful and worthy of our engagement, all coming together into a forward-looking optimism.

The concept of Sense of Coherence brings together ideas of identity and meaningfulness as espoused by Erikson and others, social cohesion as described by Barchas and Mendoza (1984) or Burch and Hamilton-Smith (1991) and the tension between individualism and community as conceptualised by Benhabib (1992). Its forward-looking optimism is very like the pleasure-centred concepts of Ornstein and Sobel in *Healthy Pleasures*. In other words, there is an emerging consensus about the importance of some sort of social integration and meaningfulness in wellness, irrespective of the words used to discuss or define it.

Finally, I return to what all this might mean in practice. At the acute (tip-of-the-iceberg) level we see the tragedy of suicide amongst young Australian males. In part, these young men face the impossibility, within their life-world, of developing a forward-looking optimism. But more profoundly, they are increasingly confronted with major disjunctions between rhetoric and reality, and the consequent difficulties in finding a meaningful sense of self which they can relate to any sort of social context. At one level, this demands a more coherent and comprehensible sense of direction in the broader society; at another, the development of a socialising society which will create meaningful opportunities for a more diverse range of life directions; and at still another, the re-establishment of adequate community support services.

But below the tip of the iceberg, a not dissimilar set of problems faces men of all ages. Cultural changes in gender roles and relationships, socioeconomic changes in the world of work, and personal changes in perceptions and expectations are all giving rise to uncertainty, stress and depression. Although the rhetoric of success through individual competitiveness drives many to a tenuous economic success and to work quite excessive hours, it drives many others to unemployment, or at least limited work opportunity and hence economic difficulty with its further impact upon family and social life. Worse still, our whole pattern of community is following the economic irrationalism of the work world; recreation is increasingly being based in commercial operation and being competitive; all too little attention is given to opportunities for social relationships, for the development of personal life-interests, or even the fostering of simple pleasure for its own sake. In this environment, it is all too easy for life to lose its meaning, and hence its immense value.

Note

This paper was originally prepared for and presented at the Conference on Men's Health Issues, convened by Bendigo Community Health Services Inc., Bendigo, Victoria, Australia, and held on 22 March 1996.

References

Antonovsky A (1979): *Health, Stress and Coping*. San Francisco: Jossey-Bass.

Antonovsky A (1987): *Unravelling the Mystery of Health: How People Manage Stress and Stay Well.* San Francisco: Jossey-Bass.

Barchas PR and Mendoza SP (eds) (1984): *Essays towards a Sociophysiological Perspective.* Westport, Connecticut: Greenwood Press.

Benhabib S (1992): *Situating the Self: Gender, Community and Post-modernism in Contemporary Ethics.* Cambridge: Polity Press.

Bolger N, DeLongis A, Kessler RC and Wethington E (1989): The contagion of stress across multiple roles. *Journal of Marriage and the Family* 51: 175–183.

Broom D (1989): Masculine Medicine, Feminine Illness: Gender and Health. In: Lupton, Gillian and Najrnan, Jake M (eds) *Sociology of Health and Illness.* Brisbane: University of Queensland Press, pp. 121–134.

Burch WR and Hamilton-Smith E (1991): Mapping a New Frontier: Identifying, Measuring and Valuing Social Cohesion Benefits Related to Nonwork Opportunities and Activities. In: Driver BL, Brown PJ and Peterson GL (eds): *Benefits of Leisure.* State College, Pennsylvania: Venture Publishing, pp. 367–380.

Caplan G (1974): *Support Systems and Community Mental Health.* New York: Behavioural Publications.

Cassel J (1976): The contribution of the social environment to host resistance. *American Journal of Epidem'ology* 104: 107–123.

Crawford J, Kippax S, Onyx J, Gault U and Benton P (1992): *Emotion and Gender.* London: Sage Publications.

Csikszentmihalyi M (1975): *Beyond Boredom and Anxiety.* San Francisco: Jossey-Bass.

Csikszentmihalyi M (1990): *Flow: The Psychology of Optimal Experience.* New York: Harper & Row.

Csikszentmihalyi M and Kleiber D (1991): Leisure and Self-actualisation. In: Driver BL, Brown PJ and Peterson GL (eds): *Benefits of Leisure.* State College, Pennsylvania: Venture Publishing, pp. 91–102.

Gibson D and Mugford S (1986): Expressive Relations and Social Support. In: Kendig H (ed.): *Ageing and Families: A Social Networks Perspective.* Sydney: Allen & Unwin.

Hamilton-Smith E (1981): The Concept of Recreational Specialisation. In: Mercer DC (ed.): *Outdoor Recreation: Australian Perspectives.* Melbourne: Sorrett.

House JS, Landis KR and Urnberson D (1988): Social relationships and health. *Science* 241: 540–545.

Lobo F (1997): Adapting to unemployment with reduced income and personal resources. *Newsletter of the International Committee on the Sociology of Leisure,* September: 14–20.

Maccoby EE (1990): Gender and relationships: A developmental account. *American Psychologist* 45: 513–520.

Miller S (1983): *Men and Friendship.* San Leandro, California: Gateway Books.

Nardi PM (1992): *Men's Friendship: Research on Men and Masculinities.* Newbury Park, California: Sage Publications.

Offe C (1985): *Disorganised Capitalism.* Cambridge: Polity Press.

Ornstein R and Sobel D (1989): *Healthy Pleasures.* Reading, Massachusetts: Addison-Wesley.

Rawlins WK (1992): *Friendship Matters: Communication, Dialectics and the Life Course.* New York: Aldine de Gruyter.

Rees S (1995): Greed and Bullying. In: Rees S and Rodley G (1995): *The Human Costs of Managerialism.* Sydney: Pluto Books, pp. 197–210.

Rook KS (1990): Social Relationships as a Source of Companionship: Implications for Older Adults' Psychological Well-being. In: Sarason BR, Sarason IG and Pierce GR (eds) (1990): *Social Support : An Interactional View.* New York: Wiley, pp. 219–250.

Stebbins RA (1992): *Amateurs, Professionals and Serious Leisure.* Montreal, Canada: McGill–Queen's University Press.

Ulrich RS, Dimberg U and Driver BL (1991): Psychophysiological Indicators of Leisure's Benefits. In: Driver BL, Brown PJ and Peterson GL (eds): *Benefits of Leisure.* State College, Pennsylvania: Venture Publishing, pp. 73–89.

Wellman B (1992): Men in Networks: Private Communities, Domestic Friendships. In: Nardi PM (1992): *Men's Friendship: Research on Men and Masculinities..* Newbury Park, California: Sage Publications.

Wright PH (1989): Gender Differences in Adults' Same- and Cross-gender Friendships. In: Adams, Rebecca G and Blieszner R (eds): *Older Adult Friendship: Structure and Process.* Newbury Park, California: Sage Publications, pp. 197–221.

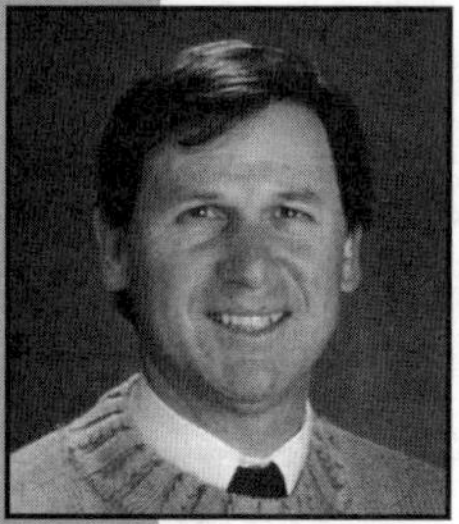

TONY EARLE

Bachelor of Education, Diploma of Teaching, Master of Education, Master of Psychology
Consultant, Earle Consultancy Services (Australia)

Tony Earle holds masters degrees in sociology (social psychology) and education (curriculum management) from the University of Missouri — Columbia, together with a Bachelor of Education and a Diploma of Teaching. His knowledge, speaking expertise and exceptional analytical skills have been sought locally and overseas by professional associations. His experiences include employment as a teacher, deputy principal and principal in schools, and as a university lecturer.

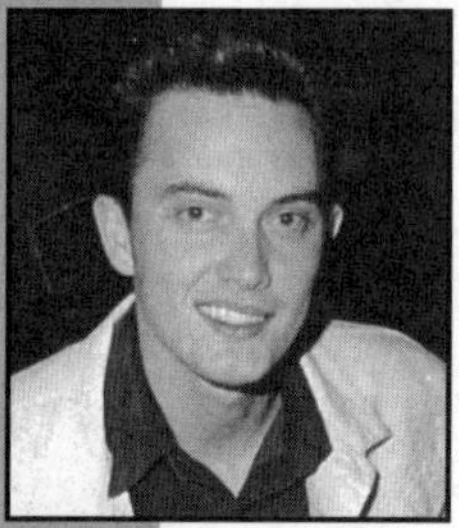

RICHARD EARLE

Bachelor of Arts
Media and Public Relations Coordinator, Earle Consultancy Services (Australia)

Richard Earle is a Bachelor of Arts graduate of the University of South Australia where he majored in media studies and community development (social policy) and completed a specialisation in communications. He has served as a university student president, branch director, activities officer, recreation officer, Media Relations Research Officer for Australia's National Seniors Association and a public relations coordinator in private and government sectors. Richard is a member of the Public Relations Institute of Australia.

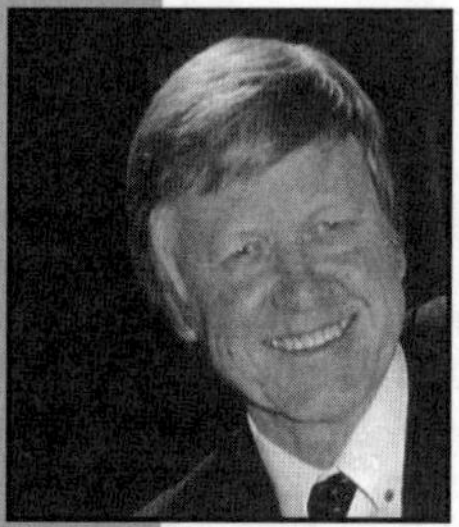

LEON EARLE

Bachelor of Arts, Master of Arts, Diploma of Teaching (Primary), Diploma of Speech and Drama, Master of Education, Doctor of Philosophy (Monash University)
Adjunct Associate Professor, Northern Territory University; Director, Earle Consultancy Services (Australia) and Earle Consultancy Services (Northern Territory)

Dr Earle was commissioned by the Minister of Ageing in South Australia to chair South Australia's Ten Year Plan on Aged Care Services and by the Minister of Health in the Northern Territory to prepare the Territory's Successful Ageing Vision Paper.

The material included in this chapter is the outcome of the authors' involvement in a national longitudinal study into successful ageing, their leadership responsibilities for the preparation of South Australia's Ten Year Plan on Aged Care Services, their part in preparing the Northern Territory's Successful Ageing Vision Paper, their aged care training and their employment with Australia's largest organisation representing older people, National Seniors.

Chapter 8

SUCCESSFUL AND HEALTHY AGEING AMONG AUSTRALIAN MEN: WINNING AND LOSING

INTRODUCTION

To group successful ageing with healthy ageing is rather complex. However, to do so can provide a useful comprehensive framework for analysis, because the two dimensions are integrated (see Figure 8.1) Research by Earle (1996) has identified six indicators of successful ageing: security, involvement, satisfaction, autonomy, integration and creativity. The first of these, security has a focus on healthy ageing while the others have a social–psychological focus. Security has two dimensions: **functional security**, which incorporates physical wellbeing (physical fitness, dexterity etc.), dietary habits, safety and finance, which collectively influence physical health; and **reflective security**, which influences mental health. Reflective security is a crucial process of personal review that follows a significant event such as withdrawal/termination from work. It is argued that, in the case of older men, the negative impact of reflective security is a mental health issue because many conduct this in comparative isolation in both interpersonal dynamics and physical setting. This may be why so many men seek the solitude and familiarity of their sheds. Reflective security also has physical health implications because a negative self-image can result in lack of personal care and a reluctance to visit health professionals. On the other hand, men who are achieving the indicators of successful and healthy ageing have a stronger inclination to preserve their health because they are enjoying life.

The social–psychological indicators of involvement, satisfaction, autonomy, integration and creativity will be discussed later in the chapter. It will be argued that successful ageing is the broader concept, so healthy ageing will be presented as a subset of successful ageing. However, the impact of the relationship between social–psychological and mental–physical wellbeing varies considerably among individuals.

Figure 8.1 Dimensions of successful/healthy ageing

INDICATORS	ORIENTATION
Security Functional Reflective	***Physical and mental health maintenance***
Involvement (in activities and interactions) ***Satisfaction*** (quality activities and interactions) ***Autonomy*** (choices) ***Integration*** (links, associations) ***Creativity*** (challenges — something to look forward to)	***Social and psychological ageing achievement***

This chapter will examine four themes:

- Who are older Australian men?
- What gender variations are there in ageing?
- Who is winning and losing in the quest to achieve the indicators of successful ageing?
- What are the implications for health and community professionals?

IDENTIFYING OLDER AUSTRALIAN MEN

In contemporary Australian society, it is no longer appropriate to link ageing to a single event such as retirement age. Today Australians are living longer and retiring earlier. In addition Australia is experiencing something of an 'age wave' with three 'mores' occurring concurrently:

More older people in good health
More older people in reasonable health
More older people in poor health

Because Australians are living longer and retiring earlier it means that planning for older people should have a focus on two crucial areas:

- community involvement options for those who are in good health; and
- community/residential/hospital care services needs for those who are not enjoying good health or who have acute care requirements (see Table 8.3 at the end of the chapter).

Table 8.1 Population projections for people aged 65 and over, 1996–2051

Projected percentages of total population and numbers							
Group	**1996**	**2001**	**2006**	**2011**	**2026**	**2031**	**2051**
Per cent	**12.0**	**12.3**	**12.9**	**14.0**	**19.3**	**20.7**	**23.1**
Number (millions)	2.204	2.385	2.6236	2.970	4.5538	5.0155	6.0306

(This table is based on ABS Series A Projection of the Population of Australian States and Territories, 1996. It is noted that there are some variations from the 1996 census figures released in 1997.)

Table 8.1 reveals that the ageing of the population is starting to accelerate and that the rate of acceleration will increase over time. In 2051, compared with 1996, there will be almost three times the number of people aged 65 and older.

With the ageing of Australia's population, it is evident that policy development for older men and women in varying degrees of health and community involvement has emerged as a major factor. It is time to identify older Australians with a more inclusive age range made up of four sectors which reflect differing characteristics, issues and needs (see Table 8.2 as a basis for policy development).

The age range incorporates:

- older aged (75 years and over)
- younger aged (65–74 years)
- emerging aged (46–64 years)
- hidden aged (35-55 years — people who are ageing prematurely)

In contemporary Australian society, older men are those in the four-sector age range who require policies or lifestyle preparation and care compensation to assist them in negotiating the quest to achieve successful and healthy ageing. This means that ageing must have a health and community need policy orientation to replace the outmoded specific retirement designation of old age. The community need age range focus must incorporate:

- contemporary longevity patterns
- work disengagement patterns
- retirement preparation

Table 8.2 Australian aged range sectors: characteristics and issues

Group identification	Characteristics	Issues
***Older aged* 75 + years**	Rapidly growing sector Varying degrees of health status Varying degrees of independence Highest need for care support Higher proportion of females than males because females live longer than males Highest care costs among females in year prior to death Men more isolated, with limited social networks	Pending shortage of quality residential centres Quality care in residential settings Community care support if living independently Care costs, assistance, access Financial changes to facilitate Ageing in Place options Community involvement options Healthy ageing needs Shortage of family carers Relocation and companionship
***Younger aged* 65–74 years**	Very rapidly growing sector Higher proportion seeking quality independent living Increasing use of community support services Higher proportion of females (except in the Northern Territory) Male reluctance to seek health care	Successful ageing links Community involvement options Relocation Care support (especially for males) Community support Elder abuse (including abuse by young kin) Functional services Lack of access to family
***Emerging aged* 45–64 years**	Very rapidly growing sector Different life experiences and therefore different expectations Varied cultural groups in large numbers with fewer children Growing numbers of early retirees (redundancy and by choice) Higher life expectancy levels than parents More working women post-2000	Healthy ageing (dietary habits, lifestyle) Community involvement for men Social network access Fewer but more mobile children Successful ageing preparation Many middle-class women seeking quality retirement lifestyle options for 20–30 years consistent with pre-retirement patterns
***Hidden aged* 35–55 years**	'Hidden' sector because their physical and/or mental condition is old for their chronological age Mainly men Display health abuse (alcohol, smoking, other substances) Low life expectancy levels Highest proportion are indigenous Australians, many are of European descent, few are of Asian descent Early dependency/care Not valued Many live itinerant lifestyle and depend on welfare/community groups	Health education High serious health care needs Early residential care access pressures Access to public accommodation Lack of social network support (few kin, abuse and neglect) Limited finance Much assistance from community groups, who support hidden aged (e.g. Alzheimer's Association, Red Cross, National Seniors and Council on the Ageing) Rehabilitation

GENDER VARIATIONS

It is argued that Australian society places a lower value on the lives of men relative to women and children. The generally held view that in the case of a disaster such as a sinking ship the women and children should be tended first illustrates this position. Men not conforming to this expectation would risk criticism.

The self-sacrificing implicit in the masculine image is worth pursuing with respect to men not caring for their health at the individual level. Relative to women, men (according to Earle, 1996) reflect a number of differences that represent considerations for health professionals.

Socialisation and societal attitudes

Compared with women, men do not place a high value on their personal health care. Women are better nurturers of their own health and the health of their children. Moreover, according to the President of the Australian Medical Association in the Northern Territory, Dr David Meadows (personal communication) women are commonly the motivation behind many men visiting doctors for check-ups and attention.

Societal values do not encourage men to seek preventative health avenues. Moreover, most men do not enjoy being questioned about their health. However, women are encouraged to monitor their own health so they are well placed to provide a health-nurturing role in the family. Work practices have traditionally placed men in more powerful and more dangerous/risky roles relative to women. This is also evident in the voluntary sector, for example, in the bushfires in New South Wales in December 1997.

Social interaction

Women speak freely about health issues and concerns with other women through their social networking avenues. Men focus more on other issues in discussions such as sport, politics, work and the economy. Consequently the health culture among women is more conducive to recognising the positive benefits of being examined or questioned in relation to health concerns and needs.

Social interaction competence and environment comfort are important in explaining precisely what an individual's concerns are with doctors and nurses. Women in general have a social and language competence advantage in talking with male or female health professionals. Many males are not so open with female or male professionals. However, a female health professional can be highly effective by recognising the reluctance of men (especially working-class men) to discuss concerns. Such health professionals compensate for this through skilful questioning. Statements like *'I'm OK'*, *'the missus said I should come but she worries too much'*, *'I've had an off day'* are not really closed statements. They are opening statements to be pursued.

Given the reluctance of many men to discuss their health concerns openly, the physical environment is an associated concern. The small confines of a formal room and the close proximity of a health professional are foreign, to working-class men in particular.

Biological variations

In Australia women live six years longer than men which prompts the question: 'Is this due solely to biological causes or a combination of biological and social causes?' Donald Cowgill (1972) argued that the biological variation should be about two years in favour of women. If so, this means that the social and work lifestyles of men represent an enormous challenge for health professionals and health educators — to change the outmoded attitudes and practices that perpetuate male health disadvantagement.

Work–leisure transition

The transition from work to nonwork (retirement) is very sudden for most men. Moreover many men tend to be poorly prepared for retirement (except in financial planning). The issues implicit in the sudden loss of a man's pivotal role, namely work, have been well documented and are especially serious in the first year after withdrawal from the workforce. According to Earle (1996) this is why many men seek the refuge of familiar territory in the form of their backyard sheds.

A crucial variation between men and women in retirement is that a male is generally expected to become more domiciled and therefore to take on more female role activities and behaviours. In a sense, for many, this constitutes a rapid transition to less relevant roles. According to research by Tony Earle (unpublished, 1997) the loss of active motivating stresses presented by the work environment for men has negative effects in retirement because the driving, and hitherto enduring, social structure of their lives is lost. For many this results in passive but highly negative stress levels, with an associated decline in motivation.

The need for retirement preparation before retirement is crucial. Planning seminars that focus only on finance do not include lifestyle messages and can produce negative outcomes because of their narrow focus.

THE INDICATORS OF SUCCESSFUL AND HEALTHY AGEING: WINNING AND LOSING

This section will outline:

- the social–psychological indicators of successful ageing
- the variations in achievement levels

- danger signals approaching retirement
- ways in which people compensate when not achieving all of the successful ageing indicators
- forms of social loss experienced

In a way, the indicators set the scene for who is winning and who is losing. Those achieving all of the indicators are winning. Those who are not heeding the danger signals and pursuing compensatory strategies are more likely to be struggling to achieve all of the indicators. Those experiencing social loss are clearly losing the quest for successful and healthy ageing.

Successful ageing — indicators

Security

Security has two main forms: functional security (personal safety; finance; dietary habits, health maintenance and access to medical and community services; mental well being); and reflective security, which takes place at a time of significant change in our lives and makes us review what has been achieved and assess both what can be carried forward and what should be done in the future to meet new needs. A negative assessment can pre-empt mental and social complexities.

Involvement

Involvement requires ongoing activities (a basis for identity) and social interactions, or people with whom we can share those activities (i.e. social support networks), which means an accessible personal community of kin and friends.

Satisfaction

Satisfaction comes from involvement in quality activities and quality interactions.

Autonomy

Autonomy implies the potential for an individual to make choices from options. This should not be regarded only as pursuing interests in isolation. We also need other people and services.

Integration

For older people integration is satisfied by sharing activities and social interactions with a range of people and doing so across several important areas such as family, leisure, religion, health and education. Economic means and personal health care are important functional considerations in this process as is access to community support services.

Creativity

Creativity implies personal challenges, for example involvement in social walking activities, with some variations such as changing the walking venue to a new location; learning new skills; doing something different and being able to discuss activities with someone.

The achievement of all these indicators is seen as essential to successful ageing. This might require adaptations to meet future needs and accessing community service organisations to pursue old and new social links and activities.

Variations in achieving the indicators of successful ageing

Gender Women tend to age more successfully than men.

Class Middle-class men tend to maintain activities but not always their social networks. Working-class men are more deficient in social networks and social activities and therefore are the major losers.

Residential location Older established areas tend to offer more services.

Community development officers Access to effective community development and recreation officers has a positive effect in connecting people to activities and social interaction possibilities.

Health-maintenance habits Women tend to speak to more people about their health and visit doctors more often. Men tend to speak only to their partners who prompt them to seek help after deferment and the risk of more serious developments. Therefore men's health is a family issue and nurses should note this.

Societal health value There is evidence that less value is placed on men's health than on the health of women and children.

Danger signals approaching retirement

The following factors present threats to the physical, mental and social health of men:

- lack of a sense of personal identity and purpose
- lack of ongoing activities from pre-retirement to retirement
- lack of access to social support networks
- carrying all work-based, stratified, partner role relationships into a partnership after retirement at the cost of companionship and sharing
- relocation after retirement without careful consideration being given to the maintenance of activity access and social support network access
- lack of personal vision and planning to meet individual (and partner) needs

- lack of personal confidence in being able to cope with changing societal values and developments
- unwillingness to visit health professionals on a regular basis

Strategies that people use to compensate for a loss of activities and interactions

People use a range of strategies to compensate for the absence of ongoing activities and friendships. These strategies will involve:

Sheds. For men sheds are like work — a place you go to and come back from; and the assumption is that a man is doing something useful while he is there! While sheds provide men with activities, they often become centres of isolation and not social centres.

Shops. Some men (and many women) go to shops for social reasons as well as to purchase goods. This means shopping centres are not just commercial centres but also social centres which could be used to facilitate learning activities, recreational pursuits etc.

The 'pokies' give people something to look forward to (but much research is needed into the long-term social effects of the pokies).

Pets serve as trusted and loyal companions but older people also require human contacts.

Talk-back radio provides live valuable interaction and information but it is vicarious rather than direct.

All of the above can be more productive if they are shared with others or at least shared in discussion.

Forms of social loss

Some men experience severe social losses if they don't achieve the elements of successful ageing. This loss is often indicated by:

- male mid-life crisis, following the loss of or a decline in a successful role
- elder abuse — usually a symptom of the vulnerability of older people in society and carer frustration
- chronic loss syndrome — perceived irretrievable social losses, activity losses and a separation from connecting agencies (higher among men than women) (Earle, 1996:97–101)
- suicide, which is commonly linked to serious personal losses (e.g. partner, home, car, shed, role, health, mobility) and intense, unbearable despair

Suggestions for ways in which men might age successfully

- It is crucial that men know the indicators of successful ageing and implement personal plans to achieve each of them (e.g. high priority for health, planning to live on retirement income the year before retirement, consulting a financial planner, maintaining activities, building new social networks).
- Because Australian men are living so much longer, they must seek involvement in work-related activities and/or nonwork-related activities such as recreation, community service and education. Starting with a personal learning journey such as writing a family history can provide motivation.
- Through education, men can learn how to operate in new areas (e.g. computers); meeting others in the process is a positive initiative.
- In the absence of kin or in the face of declining networks, older men should be encouraged to join clubs and associations representing older people (e.g. University of the Third Age (U3A), National Seniors, Council of the Ageing, Australian Retired Persons Association,) and those groups offering involvement in specific interests such as walking, cards, sports of various kinds etc.
- Pursuing activities at the local level provides a sense of familiarity. Older men should be encouraged to visit their local council and meet the community development/community service or recreation officer to find out what is available and what might be of interest.
- Men must make regular visits to health professionals to ensure that they maintain their health.

Retirement is a learning journey for older men. Indeed, like education and employment, retirement can also be hard work, requiring ongoing education and ongoing productive community involvement!

IMPLICATIONS FOR HEALTH AND COMMUNITY CARE PROFESSIONALS

Awareness of social/health need patterns

It is clear that, for older Australian men, there is a major community involvement challenge and a health services challenge. There are social realities in the lifestyle of Australian men that have negative implications for their health status and for the achievement of successful ageing.

Relative to older women older men tend to be:

- less socially flexible
- less socially competent
- less language skilled
- less willing to do new things
- less willing to leave the family home
- less willing to seek medical/health assistance
- less likely to live beyond 75 years

Many of these differences can be traced back to boyhood where not enough is done in schools to redress social/language skills deficiencies among boys.

The emerging age wave

The unprecedented increasing numbers of older people beyond 2000 will place enormous strains on social security services. Men's health must be improved through health education programs and more accommodating medical care services.

CONCLUSION

It is important that health care and community professionals:

- understand the variations between men and women and adapt their approaches accordingly
- accept as a professional obligation the imperative of advancing the status of care afforded to men
- work to provide productive community involvement options for men
- promote the importance of men accessing health services
- note that men are reluctant to discuss health difficulties with care professionals
- pursue coordination efforts across community and care dimensions
- help change the low profile given to men's health by working with public relations professionals
- encourage men approaching retirement to read literature on successful ageing patterns and needs and to attend retirement seminars that go beyond financial planning

A possible vision plan to meet the needs of older men is shown in Figure 8.2. This reveals the age range sectors, the associated need dimensions and an approach that incorporates policy development and policy coordination.

The challenge for health care and community development professionals post-2000 is to assist men to become more aware of their health and social needs and to be more responsible for them. A positive informed commitment will set the scene for a transition from what is to what can be for older Australian men.

Figure 8.2

A SUCCESSFUL Ageing Vision Plan FOR MEN

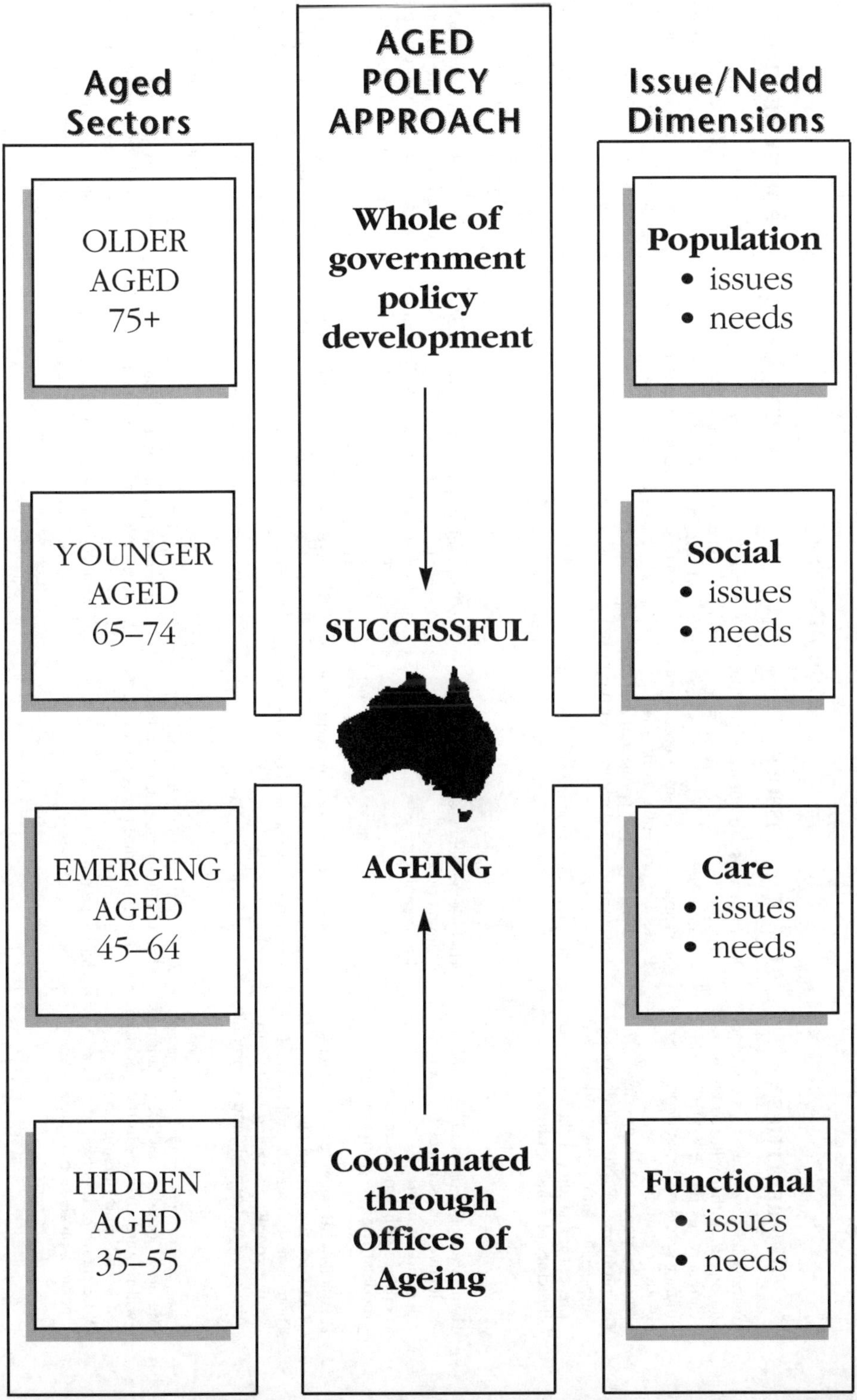

Table 8.3 Selected care dimension challenges for Australian men

CARE DIMENSION			
REALITIES	**ISSUES**	**NEEDS**	**POLICY RECOMMENDATIONS**
Australia has two major aged sectors among men that will require more care services post-2000 (because of higher levels of dependency). • Older aged 75+ • Hidden aged (premature ageing) The problems of difficult behaviour (especially among the hidden aged) present management difficulties for directors of nursing programs.	Rapid increase in numbers of older aged (75+) Isolated men Servicing costs for small communities Excessive dementia levels and substance abuse (projected increase of around 185 per cent over the next 30 years) Difficult behaviour management	Serviced residential care accommodation consistent with Ageing in Place requirements Facilities to manage/isolate difficult individuals in care centres	A coordinated collaborative plan that assesses residential care needs with plans for future role directions of existing hostels and nursing homes including: • Management of difficult behaviour of individuals • The provision of more specialised dementia facilities in chosen location(s) • A program to fight substance abuse-related dementia
There are deficiencies in established palliative care services for older dependent men. There are deficiencies in after-hours medical services in many areas.	High-dependency care service limitations Prolonging care when life quality is poor	To develop quality palliative care services Scope for directive self-determination re care Access to care	The collaborative development of palliative and care directive programs. Planned after-hours care (doctors, nurses etc.)
Hospitals offer a primary acute care focus for the community. There is a shortage of professionals with expertise in ageing relative to the need in hospitals and community care.	Servicing non-acute care requirements of older people Premature discharge processes among older people	Effective liaison re-entry and discharge of older people Provision of services for non-acute care needs More gerontologists and geriatricians	Residential care and hospital senior staff should meet to identify areas of difficulty and shortfalls in service provision and make recommendations to resolve these. Appointment of geriatricians, gerontologists, gerontological nurses
The new Commonwealth legislation will require changes in the operation of hostels and nursing homes. Older men are less likely to seek medical/professional care services.	The ability to meet structural and service requirements within stated time limits Men's health Shortage of carers	Visionary planning and collaboration Accessible services for older isolated men Attitude change and awareness raising on health care services options and their value for men Available carers	The development of a coordination strategy to identify older men in need of care, working with local doctors, health personnel, community care/support groups and Offices of Ageing.

Bibliography

Australian Bureau of Statistics (ABS) (1996): *Projection of the Population of Australian States and Territories,* Series A. Canberra: AGPS

Cowgill D (1972): Ageing and Modernisation. Unpublished paper. University of Missouri — Columbia.

Earle L (1996): *Successful Ageing in Australian Society: A Community Development Challenge.* Adelaide: Recreation for Older Adults (Australasia).

Earle L and Earle R (1997): *Northern Territory Vision Paper on Successful Ageing.* Darwin: ECS.

Edgar D, Earle L and Fopp R (1993): *Introduction to Australian Society.* Sydney: Prentice Hall.

Mather S (1997): *Aged Care Services in Australia's States and Territories.* Canberra: Australian Institute of Health and Welfare.

McCallum J (1997): Health and Ageing. Paper presented to National Geriaction Conference, Adelaide.

Personal communication

Dr David Meadows, President of the Australian Medical Association in the Northern Territory, August 1997

Section Three

MEN WITHIN THE FAMLY

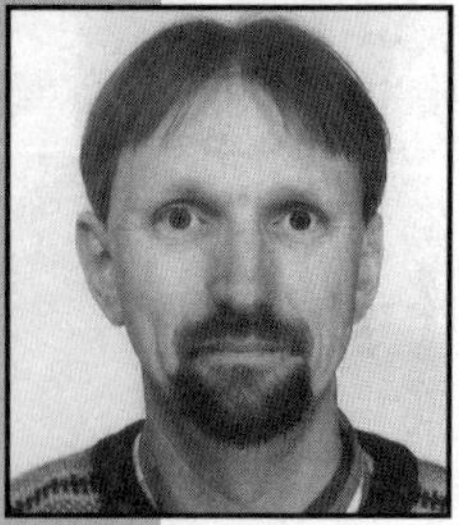

TOM LAWS

Registered Nurse, Registered Midwife, Opthalmic Nursing Diploma, Bachelor of Economics

Lecturer, Faculty of Nursing, University of South Australia

Tom Laws began his career as a registered nurse, specialising in acute care nursing and ophthalmology. After completing an Ophthalmic Nursing Diploma at Moorfields Eye Hospital in London he returned to Australia and studied midwifery. It was as a midwife that he became acutely aware of the limited knowledge that many fathers possessed in relation to childbirth and care of the mother and infant. From that point on he took a keen interest in the way men perceive, access and promote health.

A degree in economics from The University of Adelaide provided him with a basis for understanding how market forces affect the provision of health care services and how social and political forces shape the delivery and distribution of these services. He now teaches health economics to postgraduate students. His studies in the Department of Public Health at The University of Adelaide have resulted in the development of a thesis which looks at the ways and extent to which men feel they contribute to health care within the family.

Chapter 9

Men's contribution to health care within the family

Traditionally, the providers of care and health care within the family have been women. Mothers and wives have also been the interface between the family, health care providers and a variety of sources of health information. However, social change has resulted in pressure to alter or reduce these traditional roles. Women now spend more time outside the family. Since the Second World War, women's participation in the workforce has been increasing steadily as a result of part-time employment or a chosen career. As a consequence, women are faced with the choice of either adopting a dual role as carer and employee or divesting part of the caring role to other members of the family.

For men there have been:

- changes to labour markets,
- fluctuations in economic activity, and
- action by unions resulting in greater out-of-work time and leisure time.

The average time men devote to paid work fell from 50 hours per week in 1974 to 44 hours per week in 1987 (Bittman, 1992: 27). Since 1974 there has been a downward trend resulting mainly from the casualisation of labour

Although these events have increased the opportunity for men to participate in family activities and health-related matters, their ability and propensity to do so has yet to be fully assessed. Moreover, men may not have the desire to change their role within the family because that would challenge their appreciation of what it means to be masculine. There are also a number of hurdles created by society which need to be addressed by public health agencies and other health-related organisations if the transition to this new role is to be made easier and more widespread. This chapter will explore the friction that exists between traditional masculine roles and the need to expand those roles in order to maximise the health status of the family.

THE FAMILY

Any discussion pertaining to the contribution men make within the family must take into account the nature of family life. In June 1992 there were 4 775 200 families in Australia, 90 per cent of whom cared for dependent children (Briggs, 1994). These children require a wide range of care in order to develop into healthy adults. They also require surveillance by adults in order to detect signs of actual and potential health problems. If a problem is detected then an assessment should be made to establish what treatment is needed and to determine if medical intervention is required. The quality and quantity of this type of care to a large extent depends on

- the continuity of the relationship between the adults,
- their negotiated roles, and
- a sense of accountability toward the children.

The increase in family diversity in recent times has brought into question the quality and quantity of care afforded to children. In the year 1991 the parents of 46 697 Australian children were divorced. By the year 2000 it is expected that 40 per cent of all families will be the result of remarriage. A product of these remarriages is a blend of children from different parents. Added to this is an increasing trend toward cohabitative relationships involving children (Briggs, 1994). Problems regarding the detection and management of health problems in blended families of the types outlines can take many forms. For example, communication about health problems and general concern may be hindered by the nature of the relationship between adult and child. There may be resentment towards stepfathers or men cohabiting with mothers. Moreover, men marrying into a family that has been through a divorce may find it difficult to define their new role. How men cope in these situations is largely unknown. This represents a gap in current research priorities yet the magnitude of change within families is quite striking.

A number of international studies (Hantrais, 1990; Carlsen and Jorgen, 1987; Brannen, 1991) have attributed this increase in diversity to the following phenomena. Many women work outside the home as well as performing housework. These women struggle with dual roles and many are living with husbands whose roles are only slightly different from those of their fathers. That is to say, most men, particularly those working in blue-collar jobs, perceive their role as one of 'breadwinner' and are not significantly involved in joint parenting or domestic duties (Hoffman, 1989). The tensions associated with this inequality of workloads may underlay women's greater dissatisfaction with marriage than men's. Divorce rates in Australia now approach 40 per cent for first marriages and 50 per cent for second marriages and most divorce proceedings are commenced by women (Briggs, 1994).

Family breakdown does not always progress to remarriage or cohabitation. A growing number of fathers are sole parents. Solo fathers encounter some major problems in caring for their family. In the main, the attitude of the community is that single fathers cannot carry out adequately the roles traditionally assigned to women, particularly that of nurturing. Briggs believes this view is reflected in the perceived bias of the Family Court in Australia toward the mother in custody decisions. Solo fathers experience difficulties in meeting their employment and child care commitments. These problems impact on the physical and mental wellbeing of the family. Although drug abuse and even attempted suicide are cited as problems for children of solo fathers, Briggs is quick to point out that marital breakup, rather than a lack of quality care, could be associated with these difficulties (Briggs, 1994).

LINKING INCOME TO HEALTH STATUS

Men's contribution to health care within the family can, in the narrowest sense, be determined by the level of income derived from their labour. In fact, the more income and wealth in a household the better the health of individuals and families is likely to be (Smith et al., 1990). This is often attributed to healthier lifestyles and the relative ease of access to health care facilities. The ability to achieve earlier interventions in the case of illness and having the doctor or health professional of choice are also significant factors in improving health.

However, two factors work against the premise that the most effective means of promoting health care for the family is simply to work hard to secure and maintain a good wage:

1. Living on the breadline

Not all families have the level of income needed to meet all their health needs. The fact is, there are a growing number of families living on or below the poverty line for whom buying health care is just not an option.

2. It takes time to make money

To achieve higher levels of income men often spend extended periods away from the family. An analysis of contemporary work patterns (Probert, 1997) has shown that those on relatively high incomes — managers, professionals and paraprofessionals — are experiencing an increase in the intensity of work and the length of hours worked. Ironically, men in less well-paid, blue-collar occupations seem to have more opportunity to accept shorter working hours but this often reduces their total income so many seek a second job or their wives go out to work. The absence of a father and the lifestyle of dual-income families has been recognised as contributing to high levels of stress within the family and to paternal fatigue, neither of which contributes to health.

In recent years there has been an increased tendency for both parents to work. Despite the push for family-friendly workplaces:

> . . . more than a quarter of employees believe their ability to balance work and family demands has declined, and half of those who are working longer and who also have dependent children or relatives are less satisfied about this balance (Probert, 1997).

When both parents work, it is most often the mother who arranges child care and delivers and collects the child from the care centre. This may well be because many men have less flexible working arrangements. In the case where a child has to go to child care before working hours and be collected after working hours it has been estimated that the child can spend up to 12 500 hours in institutional care before starting school (NCAC, 1993).

Another reason for less time spent with the family is the increase in work availability made possible by the fax machine and the mobile telephone. These appliances have enticed men to be more available because they have ushered in a new source of social status — they provide evidence that the employee is needed and valued. To some extent, they erode traditional occupational hierarchies.

Finally, there are many men who openly admit that, after a day's work, they are not keen to return home to the emotional demands of the family and the putting to bed of children.

From the activities and behaviours outlined above it can be established that the quest for more highly paid work and, to some extent, social status leaves little opportunity for some men to contribute to health care within the family other than by the generation of income.

MEN'S CONTRIBUTION TO HEALTH CARE

Men who have gained shorter working hours or who have had them imposed are essentially an untapped resource in terms of undertaking health-related activities within the family. For the purpose of analysis these activities can be divided into **primary health care** and **secondary health care**. **Primary care** focuses on preventing disease and promoting a feeling of wellbeing. This can be achieved by activities ranging from cleaning the house and preparing a well-balanced diet to providing emotional support that defuses stress and anxiety. **Secondary health care** is concerned with restoring health once illness has occurred. It involves developing and administering treatments and monitoring for the side effects of those treatments.

Although men have the potential to contribute to the family's health and sense of wellbeing, they may be reluctant to take on this role for a number of reasons. It is widely recognised that one of the barriers to men's participation in household activities and, to a lesser extent, in caregiving revolves around the traditional gender division of labour supported by women (Holland, 1994; Merder, 1993). A study conducted by Bittman (1992), using daily diaries kept by men and women to record their paid and unpaid workloads, found that unpaid work was highly segmented into gender tasks. Male contributions to unpaid work were generally associated with traditional male activities such as home improvements or maintenance of the car, pool and yard. Although women increased the amount of paid work they did, any increases in contributions to unpaid work by men did not serve as a substitute for women's unpaid labour.

> The limited nature of men's or fathers' contribution to unpaid tasks in households with dependent children can be gauged by the fact that sole mothers have lower average unpaid work times than their parented counterparts, although they spend similar time in paid work (Bittman, 1992).

Bittman's work (using data from the Australian Bureau of Statistics) showed that, in 1974, men's contribution to household tasks was minimal. Since then men with working wives or partners have, on average, increased their participation in housework tasks by approximately two hours per week. This time is spent mostly in food preparation. Smaller increases have been noted in relation to child care, laundry and shopping (Bittman, 1992). In terms of providing child health care, men are generally reluctant to participate in the management of illness episodes. In a study by Hewison (1994) it was found that out of 282 episodes of illness, on only eight occasions was the father involved in caring. The main reason given for not participating was work commitments.

A small body of literature suggests that paid employment of the maternal partner increases parental participation by the father (Bittman, 1992). In dual-income families, more than 50 per cent of couples report an equity in performance of household tasks. However, the general consensus is that women desire men to take a more equitable role but men have been slow to take this up. In recognition of the problem the Austrian government has proposed legislation requiring men to contribute more to domestic work so as to relieve the pressure on working mothers (Lacey, 1998).

Although it would appear that gender roles are difficult to change there are men who willingly reverse roles with their partners. According to Grbich, fathers' involvement as primary caregivers is not necessarily linked to their employment status. This claim is based on a small study of 25 fathers for whom '. . . in only a small minority of cases was caregiving adopted as a result of unemployment'. In some cases the role change occurred over a number of years and was linked to some family crisis. There was also the suggestion that a father's dissatisfaction with his job could precipitate a negotiated role change with his partner (Grbich, 1994).

There is no literature available that links what men do within the family to their knowledge of primary health care. For example:

- Do men clean the toilet in the knowledge that it reduces the incidence of illness?
- Do they cook a meal on the basis that it contributes to a well-balanced diet or just to satisfy hunger?
- Do they observe their children at play and then evaluate the children's ability to reach developmental milestones?
- Do they explore their children's anxieties with a view to promoting coping strategies and a sense of wellbeing?

This last question is particularly relevant in terms of caring for the emotional wellbeing of adolescent boys who, in our society, face unclear rites of passage into manhood. One of the most touted indicators of wellbeing amongst young men is the suicide rate. Overall, males aged between 15 and 44 have a higher rate of death from suicide than do females. There has been a steady increase in youth suicide across Australia since 1960 in males but not in females. Male suicide rates are higher in nonmetropolitan areas and areas of high youth unemployment (Krupinski et al., 1994). While researchers search for causes there is little evidence to suggest that fathers are being made more aware of the warning signs exhibited by those who intend to suicide. Nor are there any strategies in place to aid men in exploring the concerns of their young sons. This may be attributed to the lower priority given to public health initiatives on mental health problems in Australia.

In the area of secondary health care there is a dearth of information to describe men's activities. For example:

- Are men able to determine if their child is sick?
- What are the criteria that men use to determine if their child requires medical intervention?
- If medications are prescribed do men know how to administer the appropriate doses safely and effectively?
- Do men know how to monitor for side effects of medications?
- What first aid skills do men possess?

Many of these questions relate to how men come by their health information. We do know that much of the information women receive is through

- health care services such as the Child and Adolescent Health Family Service (CAHFS) in South Australia and its equivalent bodies in other parts of Australia,
- antenatal and postnatal education,

- family planning centres and
- health advice contained in a plethora of women's magazines.

There are few comparable resources for men. This means that there is no substantial base from which men can acquire the knowledge and skills necessary to provide secondary health care.

RISK TAKING AND ROLE MODELLING

It is now well established that there are a number of masculinities rather than one masculine type of behaviour (Connell, 1995; Hearn, 1994). There is, however, a common element, and that is, men generally behave in ways that detract from their health status and the health status of others. This point has been made in several of the chapters in this book so does not require reiteration. What does require emphasis are the ways in which men consciously inculcate and perpetuate behaviours in the next generation of young men. The perpetuation of masculine traits that involve risk-taking behaviour may be attributed either to ignorance of the extent of the damage that can ensue or to purposeful intent.

One of the most potent sources of role modelling is sport. There is tacit agreement in our society that young boys are allowed, and at times actively encouraged by their fathers, to play sports and games that put them at higher risk of injury than young girls. Consequently, hospital records show that boys between these ages of 1 and 14 have a far higher incidence than girls of sporting injuries and other accidents caused by bumping and colliding (ABS, 1989).

Football players are idols and role models for young boys who are eager to emulate players' risk-taking behaviour on and off the field. The number of knee reconstructions needed by players of Australian rules football and the proliferation of sports injury clinics is testament to the ferocity with which men play sport.

Why do men readily allow themselves to suffer pain, injury and, possibly, disability? Research by Mildred Blaxter sheds some light on the issue:

> . . . if behaviour is unhealthy, and seemingly careless of the health consequences, it may be that it is simply not seen as relevant to health, or that the rewards outweigh any costs (Blaxter, 1995).

Put another way, many behaviours regarded as undesirable by health professionals may play an important part in the development of an individual's sense of self-worth and sense of belonging in the community. In this case, health can be seen as a means to other valued ends (being recognised as masculine) and not as an end in itself. This does not mean that the satisfaction derived by males in pursuit of masculine traits should be allowed to outweigh the health consequences. There are substantial social and economic costs incurred by the community from risk-taking activities.

This is not an argument for the prohibition of some sports but rather a reason for the development of strategies that would serve to diminish the number and severity of injuries. For example, the modification of rules in all football codes so as to reduce dangerous tackling and the compulsory use of protective equipment in contact sports could be an initial step. The element of compulsion would eliminate then any claim that those wearing safety equipment were lesser men than others on the field. In a more general sense, any sports training might include the teaching of injury minimisation strategies. How this could be orchestrated is a question for government and the sports industry.

Another salient form of role modelling takes place when young boys observe their fathers perform tasks in and around the home. Much of men's work at home involves the use of power tools, machinery, chemicals and other potentially dangerous implements. Despite substantial public health literature on the types of injuries sustained in the home and the kind of preventative measures that should be taken, there continues to be an alarming rate of injury. Between the ages of 1 and 14 boys sustain injuries from machinery, chemicals and firearms at much higher rates than do girls (ABS, 1989: 29). It may be that many of these accidents are the result of children trying to emulate their fathers' tasks in secret and unsupervised. However, the question here is, to what extent do men concern themselves with making the home environment safe for children and what priorities do they attribute to different safety issues? For example, are car seat restraints at the top of the list or is it keeping chemicals locked away? We also know very little about how well prepared men are in terms of managing children when performing traditionally male tasks. For example, do men provide children with safety glasses when showing them how to chop wood? Finally, the extent to which men model safe systems of work and use safety equipment is likely to influence the way their sons conduct themselves in the workplace.

CONCLUSION

The recent emergence of the men's health movement has drawn attention to the need for men to be informed about their health. Closely related to this awareness-raising is the need for men to recognise that they have the potential to contribute to their family's health beyond the simple generation of income. The need to contribute to family health care is demonstrated by the dual roles performed by many women and the pressure of social change on the family. Impediments to taking on this caring role include the perpetuation of masculine risk-taking behaviour and the lack of contemporary alternative role models. Despite this, much could be done in the area of public health to inform and educate men of the issues involved in family health and of strategies to improve the quality of life for their family. However, before strategies can be developed, we need to know more about how men contribute currently and where the deficits lie.

References

Australian Bureau of Statistics (ABS) (1989): *Hospital Statistics: Separations from Recognised and Private Hospitals, South Australia,* Cat. no. 4308.4. South Australian Health Commission, p. 29.

Bittman Michael (1992): *Juggling Time: How Australian Families Use Time* (2nd edn). Canberra: Australian Government Publishing Service.

Blaxter Muriel (1995): *Health and Life Styles*. Great Britain: Tavistock/Routledge, p. 148.

Brannen PM (1991): *Managing Mothers: Dual-earner Households after Maternity Leave.* Great Britain: Unwin Hyman, pp. 256–257.

Briggs F (1994): *Children and Families.* Singapore: Allen & Unwin, pp. 4–15.

Burdon BE (1993): Fathers in families; preliminary analysis (unpublished). Brisbane: Queensland University of Technology.

Carlsen S and Jorgen EL (1987): *The Equality Dilemma: Reconciling Working Life and Family Life Viewed in an Equality Perspective— The Danish Example.* Denmark: Munksgaard.

Connell RW (1995): *Masculinities.* Great Britain: Allen & Unwin, pp. 71–72.

Grbich C (1994): Women as primary breadwinners in families where men are primary caregivers. *Australian and New Zealand Journal of Sociology* 30 2, August: 105–118.

Hafner RJ (1986): *Marriage and Mental Illness.* USA: The Guildford Press, pp. 37–39.

Hantrais L (1990): *Managing Professional and Family Life: A Comparative Study of British and French Women.* Great Britain: Dartmouth, pp. 152 and 161.

Hearn J (1994): Research in men and masculinities: Some sociological issues and possibilities. *Australian and New Zealand Journal of Sociology* 30 1, April: 47.

Hewison J and Dowswell T (1994): *Child Health Care and the Working Mother: The Juggling Act.* Great Britain: Chapman & Hall.

Hoffman WL (1989): Effects of maternal employment in the two parent family. *American Psychologist* 44 2, February: 283–292.

Holland A (1994): Fathers and children: Dismantling the barriers to men's participation in child rearing. Paper presented at the *Issues in Australian Childhood Conference,* 23–25 September. Brisbane.

Krupinski J, Tiller J, Burrows D and Hallenstein H (1994): Youth suicide in Victoria: A retrospective study. *The Medical Journal of Australia* 160, February: 113–116.

Lacey H (1998): Equality street blues. *Independent on Sunday,* 1 March, p. 21.

Merder HJ (1993): Division of labour in two-earner homes. *Journal of Marriage and the Family* 55: 133–145.

National Childcare Accreditation Council (1993): *Putting Children First: Quality Improvement Handbook.*

Probert B (1997): Long day's journey leaves workers jaded. *Age,* 27 October: A11.

Smith D, Bartley M, Blane D (1990): The black report on socioeconomic inequalities in health 10 years on. *British Medical Journal* 301 August: 18–25.

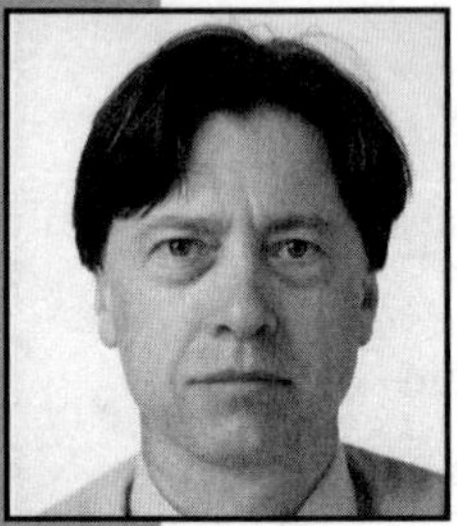

CLIVE SKENE

Bachelor of Arts, Diploma of Applied Psychology, Master of Psychology
Coordinator, Community Mental Health, Department of Public Health, Flinders University, South Australia

Clive Skene is a clinical psychologist with 13 years' experience of working with families, children and adolescents with behavioural, social and emotional problems. Nine of those years were spent at the Women's and Children's Hospital in Adelaide, South Australia, and four were in private practice.

Clive has been interested in the area of fatherhood and men's health issues since 1991.

Chapter 10

HEALTHY FATHERHOOD

There is no doubt that an ongoing adjustment is occurring within the Australian family[1] to the substantial social and economic forces currently at play. The changing face of the family in the 1980s and 1990s has, by necessity, involved changes to the previously defined roles of both mothers and fathers. However, as Paltiel (1989), Wigg (1994), Jacobs (1995) and others have maintained, the study of fatherhood has lagged far behind the research-based theory of motherhood. This is because, they argue, the agenda has mainly been set by male researchers who have consciously or subconsciously chosen to focus upon the mother–child relationship.

There has been considerable debate amongst researchers and theorists about whether or not fatherhood as a 'social institution' or 'condition' is in a state of crisis (see Knijn, 1995, and de Singly, 1995, for contrasting arguments). Some have argued that gender roles in general, but for fathers in particular, are in a deep state of crisis as Western culture moves closer to a state of androgyny (Knijn, 1995). The authority previously ascribed to the father role is said to have dissipated with the disappearance of separate Father and Mother roles. It is also argued that the current norm within families is for an equalisation of roles, where the adult male and female, undertake 'parenting' rather than gender-specific roles (Kraemer, 1991)

Factors impacting upon this blurring of gender identity include:

- an increasing emphasis on feminism in its various forms,
- the movement of more and more women into the workplace,

- high rates of unemployment (particularly amongst unskilled males), and
- advances in reproductive technology, which have effectively placed the power of procreation in the hands of the mother.

All of these factors have all contributed to the current profile of the Australian family (Deech, 1993; Marsiglio, 1995).

Other authors have argued, that although change is certainly occurring across a wide range of issues related to gender and family structure issues, this does not constitute a crisis (de Singly, 1995) Rather it is part of a continuous evolutionary process. Hareven (1995) reminded us of the need to keep current changes in a historical perspective. Viewed from a historical perspective, the two-parent nuclear family of the 1950s and 1960s (with the mother as homemaker and the father as breadwinner) represents just another phase in family development and should not be regarded as a normative structure. We should not project the isolated nuclear family image too far backwards in time when looking at change.

Hareven incorporated an historical perspective into her analysis. She believes that confusion over the expected role of fathers was also common in the 19th century. Moreover, current circumstances are part of an ongoing process rather than one of a series of 'crises'. However, it is true that previous generations of fathers were much less 'lonely' in their role. Because of closer family ties, they often had the ongoing support of their own father, uncles and grandfather(s). Larger families also meant 'surrogate' parenting by older siblings. Finally, Hareven pointed out that class issues are very important: there is greater continuity of the fatherhood role across pre-industrial and industrial working-class families than in upper-class or middle-class families.

Many studies have attempted to research the form and meaning of fatherhood by examining what they consider to be important variants of family structure, for example: sole-parent families (Wilson, 1990; Hanson, 1981), absent-father families (Rose, 1992; Gabel, 1992), stepfamilies (Mekos, Hetherington and Reiss, 1996) or same-sex-couple families (Bozett, 1989). These approaches often seek to illuminate the still-predominant family form, that is, the two-parent family unit, by examining the exceptions rather than the rule. Many of these studies have provided insights into different family forms but it seems to this author that greater benefit is derived from studying the phenomenon itself rather than seeking to derive conclusions from exceptions or analogous circumstances.

Before researchers can examine the changing nature of fatherhood within the family it is desirable to establish how society currently conceives of and constructs the role of father. Part of that social construction process is the feedback received by both mothers and fathers about what constitutes appropriate fathering. Feedback is received from a range of sources including professionals who are cast in the mould of 'expert'. These experts can include a range of health and mental health workers such as nurse therapists, community health workers, psychologists and social workers.

A social constructionist view maintains that the beliefs of individuals about their world are socially constructed; that is, they result from the 'knowledge' gained from the interpretations by themselves and others of their social interactions. 'Knowledge' is not defined in objective or empirical terms but rather as 'what people "know" as "reality" in their everyday lives.' (Berger and Luckmann, 1966:27)

Such 'knowledge', although individually acquired, also has a common or shared quality because of the social nature of its transmission. The individual experiences the 'self' within the context of an ongoing interchange with others (Bruner, 1986). If sufficient numbers of a social group have similar views then this element of their understanding may attain the status of 'commonsense knowledge'. Commonsense knowledge is described by Cuff and Payne (1989:153) as 'the knowledge of the everyday world which social actors possess by virtue of living in and being part of that world'. In other words it is 'knowledge' which is taken for granted and is rarely reflected upon in conscious awareness, as opposed to the consciously articulated parts of an ideologically based statement. An example of this 'knowledge' might be that mothers are biologically predisposed to be more nurturant than fathers or that it is 'normal' for fathers to take the role of disciplinarian within the family.

When the social constructionist perspective is adopted within a research context it may be regarded by some as unscientific. However others argue that

> . . . scientific knowledge is in large part an invention or development rather than an imitation (of reality); concepts, hypotheses, and theories are not found ready-made in reality but must be constructed.' (Diesing, 1971, quoted in Strauss and Corbin, 1991:59)

NURSING LITERATURE

Significant contributions to the growing literature on aspects of fatherhood have come from authors with a background in nursing. Part of the interest in this area appears to have been generated by a desire to explain the part played by fathers during pregnancy (Sherwen, 1986; Tiller, 1991; Conner and Denson, 1990; Jordan, 1990; Glazer, 1989; Battles, 1988), childbirth (Chapman, 1991; Bedford and Johnson, 1988; Palkovitz, 1988), and the early life of the neonate (Ferketich and Mercer, 1989; Fishbein, 1990; Fawcett, 1989). Other authors have investigated the impact on fathers of *couvade* syndrome (Longobucco and Freston, 1989) and breast-feeding (Jordan and Wall, 1990; Jordan, 1986). One of the strongest areas of interest has been the measurement of attachment or 'father–infant bonding' (Novak, 1990; Schodt, 1989; Mercer et al., 1988; Fortier, 1988). The preoccupations of professionals who work intimately with people at the time when fatherhood effectively commences should be no surprise. Neither should the focus of their investigations, despite some criticism of research in areas such as attachment/bonding theory (Palkovitz, 1988). However, nursing research has also broadened its field of interest to encompass areas such as adolescent fathers (Anderson, 1990; Castiglia, 1990; Sachs, Poland and Giblin, 1990).

FATHERHOOD AND SOCIAL CHANGE

By the 1970s social and cultural factors had changed sufficiently for men to be encouraged to become participants in, rather than distant spectators of, the arrival of their offspring. The traditional images of the expectant fathers waiting room, with its stereotypical anxious, cigarette-puffing, first-time father and his more blasé counterpart, the 'been-there done-that' multiple parent, were replaced by the 'breathing coach' and, eventually, the 'clamp and cut the cord' birthing assistant. How many men willingly chose this option and how many were reluctantly coerced into the fascinating but frightening realm of hitherto women's business remains open to speculation. However, in the space of the last twenty years, active participation in birthing by fathers has changed from unwelcome intrusion to unspoken expectation. Of course increased involvement in the birthing process is no guarantee that a father will be recognised as a carer in his own right. It may be worth asking the question: in order for fathers to have a happy and healthy relationship with their children, do they need to be recognised as having a discrete caregiving role rather than being seen as a support to the 'real' parenting of the mother?

The recognition that men can become deeply emotionally involved with their children from birth and even 'in utero' (Schodt, 1989) has contributed to their emerging emotional freedom. The freedom offered to men has been accelerated by virtue of the social and cultural changes outlined earlier. Feminism, for example, also meant 'liberation' for men from restrictive fathering roles and the opportunity to embrace participatory parenting. Critical to this point however is the degree to which men were limited by the social and familial pressures that sometimes restrict the perception and choices of the individual. It could be argued that access to the opportunity to take on a different role construction is restricted to those who can embrace a particular view of masculinity without encountering opposition from spouse, friends or extended family. Certainly those men who were not aware of these opportunities for change were not likely to have moved from the confines of their traditional role. The extent, speed and perhaps even desirability of change was subject to debate in various forums but the direction of change was unquestionably clear.

Society is obviously not a static environment although change occurs at different rates. At times it appears breathtakingly fast and may perhaps be labelled as a period of 'crisis', as discussed above. Stability could be viewed as a virtue in this context. It is seen as providing predictability and comfort. However, men in general, and fathers in particular, have suffered from a presumption by others that they are almost universally opposed to changes in family power relationships and childcare responsibilities. In fact, some men are expressing positive reactions to changing roles either by choice or necessity and are knocking on the door to enter the realm of concerned and participative parenting. It has been the 'institutional public processes' (Edgar and Glezer, 1992) associated with the family — such as government policy, employment conditions, child-care provisions and the conservative attitudes of professionals, employers and sections of the community — which have failed to let them in.

WHAT DO PROFESSIONALS SAY?

As part of a recent study conducted by the author[2] a group of ten therapists employed by a nongovernment organisation (NGO), who worked directly with families in the home, were asked to form a nondirective focus group to explore their ideas about fatherhood. Content analysis of their discussion revealed a strong emphasis upon traditional ideas about fatherhood. They described the role of fathers as *'still expected to be the breadwinner'*, *'the person who would look after the family'*, *'the protector of the family'* and *'the one who keeps everything going'*. They also viewed the father as *'usually the disciplinarian or seen to be'*. Even on the lighter side of family life they saw fathers as still the ones *'. . . playing with the kids, doing the rough and tumble with the kids, taking them fishing'*. There was some recognition of a changing society because of high levels of unemployment which resulted in *'role reversals'* where the father *'might be the caring person, getting the child ready for school, for his bath and that sort of stuff'*. However, the general consensus of their views appeared to be that fathers were and are still closely identified with traditional roles within nuclear families. The fact that a situation where a man performed the home nurturing role and the woman went out to work was still described as a reversal of roles reflects an attitude suggestive of the view that gender roles are still rigidly defined.

WHAT DO FATHERS SAY ?

Thirty-one fathers with at least one child attending a primary school, volunteered to participate in nondirective focus groups to discuss the topic of fatherhood. To avoid bias in the study the fathers were selected from schools chosen at random. Three focus groups of approximately ten fathers each were formed. One of the most striking aspects of the groups was the level of emotional release gained by the participants as the discussion progressed. The groups were clearly defined to all participants as venues for an open discussion of family issues. There was no implication that any form of therapeutic intervention would be offered. Yet in each of the groups men appeared to experience strong emotional responses to the topics discussed. This was particularly noted in discussions about men's experiences with their own fathers. Most men reported either a strong negative or a strong positive reaction to recollections of their childhood experiences of being fathered. This emotion was reflected in their behaviour, with some men becoming tearful and others expressing anger.

My own father died three years ago. It was like having my legs cut away. It was a very dramatic period in my life. We were very close right from the start. (Craig)

I feel that I missed out with my own father. He was always too busy to give any time to me. I promised myself that I would try hard to get close to my own children. I don't want them to have the same opinion of me as I have of my father. (Steve)

Other men became distressed when they recalled the 'loss' of their children as a result of separation or divorce. Although these children were not lost in the sense that formal visitation rights were denied, the common experience was the loss of the opportunity to be a family with those children. A commonly expressed view among these men was that they felt an acute need to start another family in order to experience fatherhood within the context of family life. Fatherhood outside the context of a family, although viewed as important, was not as satisfying as the experience of being part of the family unit.

I've already lost one family and it's been horrible. I'm not going to risk losing another one. So if I've got to do the housework or whatever then I'll do it. In any case it's only fair to share the load in the family. (Peter)

The most animated discussion amongst the participants in the focus groups centred around the definition of the current role fathers fulfil within the family unit. There was a strong level of dissonance in many men's minds between traditional role definitions and those implied by social changes. For some men this impacted significantly upon their ability to maintain stable self-perceptions of the meaning of fatherhood.

I've often asked myself, are men cut out to look after kids? Shouldn't we just stick to traditional roles of being breadwinner and bad guy? (Tony)

You're told to discipline the kids by the wife then you get told off by her for raising your voice — you're in the doghouse with everyone. I think most men don't know what they're supposed to be like any more. Women's roles are much clearer. (Mike)

Other men appeared to take refuge from their confusion by adhering to rigid traditional values.

Really, when it boils down to it, you're the head of the family anyway and the buck stops with you. You're the one out in the world, you've got to take the brunt of the responsibility for what goes on in the family. (Gerry)

However the predominant mood of the groups is probably best reflected by the following statement.

I wish somebody had shown me or given me some insight into how to handle the situation [of fatherhood]. *If you don't get it from your father you just run around falling over yourself, making mistakes and you get up and fall down again. Kids are always willing to love you and you can share in a lot that they do. But it doesn't stop there, you have to get involved with all the family and it's difficult. I'm finding it tremendously difficult.* (Steve)

Some of these comments could be interpreted as support for the view that fatherhood is indeed in a state of crisis. Undoubtedly these men were expressing their uncertainty and confusion. However, they were also working hard to overcome the issues that family and society caused them to confront.

They agreed that the reason they had wanted to attend the focus group was to learn how to become a better father rather than just to complain about how difficult some aspect of being a parent was for them. If this is a common view among a substantial number of fathers who cross the path of health professionals then we may indeed have the basis for significant influence upon a hitherto neglected aspect of family development. The added bonus in this equation is that, as well as enhancing their fathering ability, men who are able to resolve these issues are more likely to reduce their ongoing stress levels and enhance their emotional wellbeing as well.

EIGHT DIMENSIONS OF FATHERHOOD

Content analysis of the fathers focus group discussion suggested eight main areas or dimensions of interest and concern. These were:

1. Employment-related issues, e.g. how to 'switch off' from work problems at home and relate to the family in a positive way
2. Personal/emotional issues, such as gaining personal space to attend to your individual needs without feeling guilty about not putting the family first
3. Relationship with father — of special concern if the relationship had not been positive
4. Role-definition, particularly lack of clarity about father and mother roles and frustration with mixed messages about role expectations
5. Masculinity issues — frustration again about the perception of mixed messages such as 'be responsible for discipline but be soft and caring' and 'be the family figurehead but share the decision-making'
6. Benefits of fatherhood — expressions of emotion and pride about the joys of sharing in the lives of their children
7. Social changes and their effect on parenthood, particularly changes in society's 'appreciation' of the efforts men make as fathers
8. Developmental changes in children as they grow, e.g. disappointment when, as they near adolescence, children start to lose interest in previously close relationships with their fathers

These dimensions are not offered as definitive descriptors of fatherhood or as a model of Australian fathering issues in the 1990s. Rather they offer some insight into the issues that men are currently struggling with in order to fulfil the position of father in society.

CLINICAL PRACTICE

The genesis of the author's attempt to understand contemporary fatherhood was rooted in the clinical experience of therapeutic work in a Child and Adolescent Mental Health Service. The passing parade of clients consisted almost exclusively of children or adolescents and their mothers. Fathers were either absent from the initial consultation process or were passively and sometimes openly aggressive (verbally) to the therapist. This type of behaviour was directed predominantly towards young female therapists who were not parents. Interventions were sometimes challenged and sometimes sabotaged, overtly or covertly. Fathers often attended for one or two sessions then did not return. Insight into such behaviour, by the author and his colleagues, was only indicative of possible causes.

The above research suggests that many men are currently confused, frustrated and uncertain about their position within the family. When a parent decides that a family member requires the help of a mental health professional it is, at the very least, a tacit admission of failure to resolve a significant problem. Men who feel that their role (and perhaps their perceived status as the parent with ultimate responsibility for the wellbeing of the family) is already under threat may feel even more compromised by this admission and by the need to seek the support of an 'expert' outside the family. However, the research also suggests that many men are eagerly seeking greater clarity and understanding in this area of their lives. Sometimes all it takes is for someone to ask them, to offer a forum for the man to voice his own issues about his lived experience as a father. An expression of understanding about the social ambiguities surrounding present constructions of fatherhood can be beneficial.

SUMMARY

In this chapter I have argued that much confusion exists among both therapeutic workers and their client population about the current status, role and function of men as fathers. Some workers retained concepts involving fathers as family figurehead, protector and disciplinarian despite being aware of significant changes in the social environment. The fathers themselves, however, were increasingly questioning a social process by which their previously known roles were being 'de-constructed' without a clearly defined set of replacement expectations. Fathers, especially those who were strongly committed to their responsibilities within the family, were nevertheless struggling to come to terms with many aspects or dimensions of their lived experience of fatherhood. Acknowledging the fact that men are engaged in a difficult process of redefining and reconstructing fatherhood and offering them an opportunity to explore their reactions to the changes inherent in the process may go a long way towards enhancing therapeutic engagement. Further research is underway to assist in defining a research-based model of healthy fatherhood.

Notes

1. This chapter refers to fathers within the context of families of white, Anglo-Saxon background. To write about the complexities of cultural influences on fatherhood across the range of ethnicities represented in Australian society would require greater scope than is possible here. Readers are referred to works such as Storer, D (ed.) (1985) *Ethnic Family Values in Australia*, published in Sydney by Prentice-Hall.

2. Skene C, Unpublished PhD thesis 'Fatherhood in theory: psychological aspects of the social construction of the male parenting role in Australian family systems'. In preparation.

References

Anderson N (1990): Pregnancy resolution decisions in juvenile detention. *Archives of Psychiatric Nursing* IV 5, October: 325–331

Battles RSB (1988): Factors influencing men's transition into parenthood. *Neonatal Network* April 63–66.

Bedford VA and Johnson N (1988): The role of the father. *Midwifery* 4: 190–195

Berger P and Luckmann T (1966): *The Social Construction of Reality*. Harmondsworth: Penguin.

Bozett FW (1989): Gay fathers: A review of the literature. *Journal of Homosexuality* 18 1–2:137–62.

Bruner J (1986): *Actual Minds, Possible Worlds*. Cambridge: Harvard University Press.

Castiglia PT (1990): Adolescent fathers. *Journal of Pediatric Health Care* 4 6, November–December: 311–313.

Chapman L (1991) Searching: Expectant fathers' experiences during labor and birth. *Journal of Perinatal Neonatal Nursing* 4 4: 21–29.

Conner GK and Denson V (1990): Expectant fathers' response to pregnancy: Review of literature and implications for research in high risk pregnancy. *Journal of Perinatal Neonatal Nursing* 4 2: 33–42.

Cuff EC and Payne GCF (eds) (1989): *Perspectives in Sociology*. London: Unwin Hyman.

Deech R. (1993): The rights of fathers: Social and biological concepts of parenthood. In: Getelaar J and Sarcevic P (eds): *Parenthood in Modern Society*. Dordrecht: Martinus Nijhoff Publishers.

de Singly F (1995): Implementing a New Model of Paternity. In: Van Dongen M, Frinking G and Jacobs M (eds): *Changing Fatherhood: A Multidisciplinary Perspective*. Amsterdam: Thesis Publishers.

Edgar D and Glezer H (1992): A man's place? Reconstructing family realities. *Family Matters* 31 April: 36–39.

Fawcett J (1989): Spouses' experiences during pregnancy and the postpartum: A program of research and theory development. *Image: Journal of Nursing Scholarship* 21 3, Fall: 149–52.

Ferketich SL and Mercer RT (1989): Men's health status during pregnancy and early fatherhood. *Research in Nursing and Health* 12: 137–148.

Fishbein EG (1990): Predicting paternal involvement with a newborn by attitude towards women's roles. *Health Care for Women International* 11: 109–115

Fortier JC (1988): The relationship of vaginal and cesarean births to father–infant attachment. *Journal of Obstetric, Gynaecology and Neonatal Nursing* March–April: 128–134.

Gabel S (1992): Behavioural problems in sons of incarcerated or otherwise absent fathers: The issue of separation. *Family Process* September 31 3: 303–14.

Glazer G (1989): Anxiety and stressors of expectant fathers. *Western Journal of Nursing Research* 11 1: 47–59.

Hanson S (1981): Single custodial fathers and the parent–child relationship. *Nursing Research* 30 4, July–August.

Hareven T (1995): Comment on Yvonne Knibiehler. In: Van Dongen M, Frinking G and Jacobs M (eds): *Changing Fatherhood: A Multidisciplinary Perspective.* Amsterdam: Thesis Publishers.

Jacobs M (1995): The Wish To Become a Father: How Do Men Decide in Favour of Parenthood? In: Van Dongen M, Frinking G and Jacobs M. (eds): *Changing Fatherhood: A Multidisciplinary Perspective.* Amsterdam: Thesis Publishers.

Jordan PL (1986): Breastfeeding as a risk factor for fathers. *Journal of Obstetric, Gynaecology and Neonatal Nursing* March–April: 94–97.

Jordan PL (1990): Laboring for relevance: Expectant and new fatherhood. *Nursing Research* 39 1, January–February: 11–16.

Jordan PL and Wall VR (1990): Breastfeeding and fathers: Illuminating the darker side, *Birth* 17 4, December: 210–213.

Knijn T (1995): Towards Post-Paternalism? Social and Theoretical Changes in Fatherhood. In: Van Dongen M, Frinking G, and Jacobs M (eds): *Changing Fatherhood: A Multidisciplinary Perspective.* Amsterdam: Thesis Publishers.

Kraemer S (1991): The origins of fatherhood: An ancient family process. *Family Process* 30, December: 377–392.

Longobucco DC and Freston MS (1989): Relation of somatic symptoms to degree of paternal-role preparation of first-time expectant fathers. *Journal of Obstetric, Gynaecology and Neonatal Nursing* November–December: 482–488.

Marsiglio W (1995): Artificial Reproduction and Paternity Testing: Implications for Fathers. In: Van Dongen, M., Frinking, G. and Jacobs, M. (eds.) *Changing Fatherhood: A Multidisciplinary Perspective.* Amsterdam: Thesis Publishers.

Mekos D, Hetherington EM and Reiss D. (1996): Sibling differences in problem behaviour and parental treatment in nondivorced and remarried families. *Child Development,* October 67 5: 2148–65.

Mercer RT, Ferketich S, May K, DeJoseph J and Sollid D (1988): Further exploration of maternal and paternal fetal attachment. *Research in Nursing and Health* 11: 83–95.

Novak JC (1990): Facilitating nurturant fathering behavior in the NICU. *Journal of Perinatal Neonatal Nursing* 4 2: 68–77.

Palkovitz R (1988): Sources of father–infant bonding beliefs: Implications for childbirth educators. *Maternal–Child Nursing Journal* Summer 17 2: 101–13.

Paltiel FL (1989): Child-rearing: a task for fathers as well as mothers. *World Health Forum* 10: 249–257.

Rose MK (1992): Elective single mothers and their children: The missing fathers. *Child and Adolescent Social Work Journal* 9 1, February: 21–33.

Sachs BA, Poland ML and Giblin PT (1990): Enhancing the adolescent reproductive process: Efforts to implement a program for black adolescent fathers. *Health Care for Women International* 11: 447–460.

Schodt CM (1989): Parental–fetal attachment and couvade: A study of patterns of human–environment integrality. *Nursing Science Quarterly* 2 2, Summer: 88–97.

Sherwen LN (1986): Third trimester fantasies of first-time expectant fathers. *Maternal–Child Nursing Journal* 15 (3) Fall: 153–70.

Strauss A and Corbin J (1991): *Basics of Qualitative Research: Grounded Theory Procedures and Techniques.* Newbury Park, California: Sage.

Tiller CM. (1991): Assessment of the potential for maladaptive parenting in expectant fathers with the adult–adolescent parenting inventory (AAPI). *Journal of Child and Adolescent Psychiatric and Mental Health Nursing* 4 2, April-June: 55–61.

Wigg N (1994) *The Adelaide Advertiser.* Thursday, 7 April: 22.

Wilson J (1990): *Single fathers: Australian men take on a new role.* Melbourne: Sun Books.

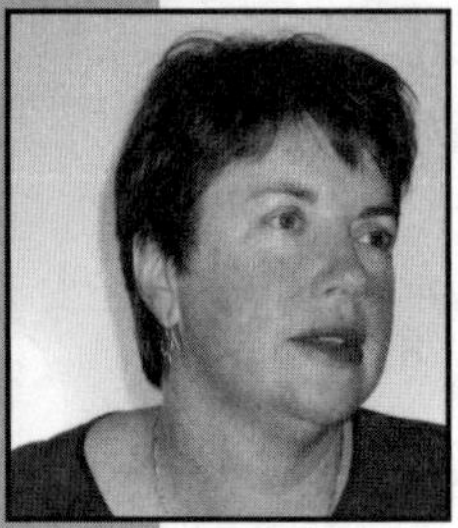

JENNY DONOVAN

Registered Nurse, Registered Midwife, Certificate of Maternal and Child Health, Bachelor of Nursing, Master of Science (Primary Health Care), Fellow of the Royal College of Nursing, Australia

Jenny Donovan is a member of The Flinders University School of Nursing in South Australia. She wrote the following notes about this chapter:

The project for my Master of Science degree evolved from the work of Barclay (1993) who interviewed couples during pregnancy and found a mismatch with regard to the sexual interest levels between men and women during pregnancy. I worked with Professor Lesley Barclay for my project and my novice research skills improved within the culture of a research-oriented and collaborative team of nurses, midwives and doctors at Flinders University. That environment provided the opportunity to develop my project within a network of skilled support and positive interest which gave me direct access to statisticians and political and professional support that would otherwise have been unavailable. The process facilitated my successful application for research funds (the project was funded by a Flinders University URB grant) and was part of a concerted and strategic effort to bring practitioners and researchers together in a nonjudgmental yet rigorously demanding environment. Regular research meetings were held involving researchers at all levels of competence undertaking numerous projects and openly sharing their research proposals and work in progress. Constant feedback on draft after draft improved our processes. This environment facilitated group learning about various research methodologies, brought diverse disciplines together and provided the support and encouragement necessary to take the next step, whether it be, for example, defending one's own project at an ethics committee meeting or discussing the difficulties surrounding recruitment. This model of research is to be highly recommended.

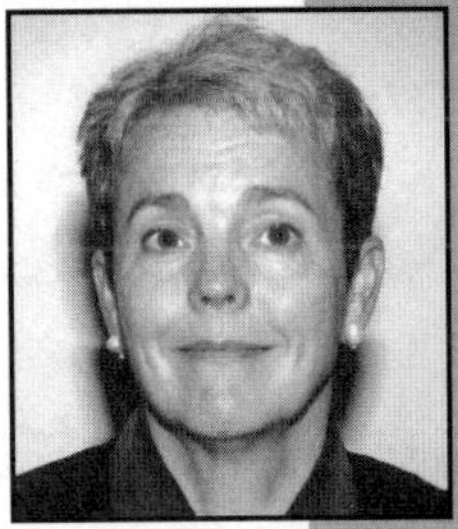

LESLEY BARCLAY

Registered Nurse, Registered Midwife, Bachelor of Social Science, Bachelor of Education, Doctor of Philosophy
Professor of Health in the Faculty of Nursing at the University of Technology, Sydney and the South Eastern Sydney Health Service

Lesley Barclay has worked as a clinician, a hospital educator, a lecturer in health education and an education officer for the Family Planning Association of Australia. She has held academic positions from lecturer to professor. Her doctoral research was into sexuality and pregnancy. Her research and writing is focused upon parenting, midwifery, family health, women in development, safe motherhood and sexuality. At present she is leading research teams funded by the National Health and Medical Research Council and the Australian Research Council studying parenting and care in nurseries that help parents attach to their children.

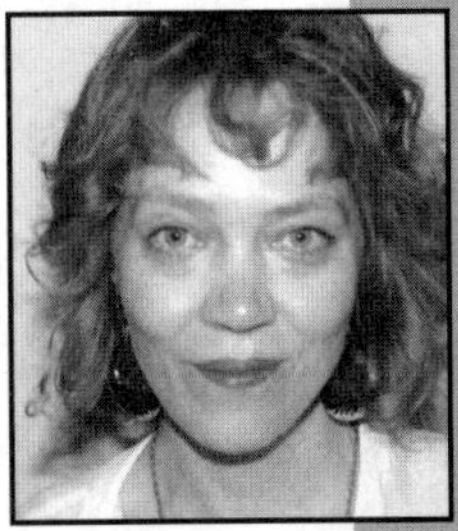

JO ENGLAND

Bachelor of Arts (Psychology), Graduate Diploma of Education, Graduate Diploma of Counselling
School Counsellor and Intern Psychologist with the Department of Education and Training in New South Wales

Jo England's work reflects a combination of her initial experience in the theatre and her subsequent involvement with education, training, research and counselling. Jo has directed actors for experiential learning in behavioural medicine, education and drug and alcohol counselling. She has also spent time working with Dr Andrew Ramsay providing clinical training programs for general practitioners. Jo's present work involves working with families. She welcomes the opportunity, provided by this chapter, to support men in redefining and developing their roles in the family — she has two sons who may become fathers!

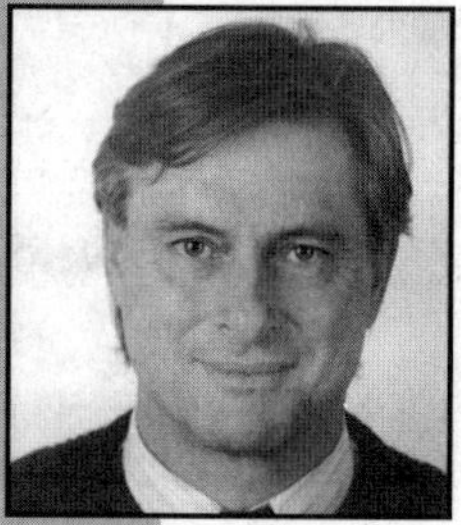

ANDREW RAMSAY

Bachelor of Medicine, Bachelor of Surgery, Diploma of Obstetrics, Member of the Royal College of Gynaecologists, Fellow of the Royal Australian College of General Practice
General Practitioner, Crafter Medical Centre, Hawthorn, South Australia

As well as working as a general medical practitioner in an Adelaide suburban practice, Andrew Ramsay is a part-time clinical tutor at The Flinders University Medical School. He has had a long association with obstetric care and was active in the areas of home birth and the development of midwife-centred care in South Australia. Andrew began conducting discussion groups for new and prospective parents in the 1970s and has continued this practice on and off to this day. Working as a member of the medical staff of a behavioural medicine clinic held weekly at Flinders Medical Centre led Andrew to a focus on counselling in his general medical practice and he currently conducts two half-day sessions a week devoted fully to counselling care.

Chapter 11

Men's transition to parenthood

INTRODUCTION

Terry (1991:527) states that

> the transition to pregnancy is one of the sharpest changes that takes place in most people's lives.

Men and women enter the transition to parenthood as a couple. However, they have arrived at this point via different pathways, that is through their childhood and their own experience of being parented, from which they have learned that there are 'rules' that state how men and women should behave (male and female stereotypes) (Cowan et al., 1985). Belsky et al. (1986) agree that the transition to pregnancy requires a restructuring of family life, and while that restructuring occurs, there is a multiplicity of pressures with which to contend. Other writers support the notion that 'the male generally has even less freedom to explore the excitement and potential growth inherent in pregnancy than does his female counterpart' (Colman and Colman, 1971:97) and that men take on new roles during pregnancy and parenthood which call for 'integration and readjustment' (Entwisle and Doering, 1981:12). When this occurs there is the possibility of role 'strain or incompatibility' (Entwisle and Doering 1981:12) which has to be negotiated within the relationship and family life.

As a means of furthering the study of men's transition to parenthood, and exploring their experiences, in 1995, Donovan, a nursing lecturer at The Flinders University of South Australia, and Ramsay, a well-known medical practitioner from South Australia, held antenatal experiential sessions with a group of six men, and Donovan, alone, held individual interviews with the men postnatally. Up until that time, little was known about the social and emotional experiences of men during their first pregnancy with their partner.

THE THEORY

Grounded theory was the chosen method of research. Grounded theory, a qualitative approach, incorporates a number of distinct features:

- Specific sampling and data collection techniques and processes used in analysis ensure rigour and comprehensiveness.
- Constant comparisons and the use of a coding paradigm ensure conceptual development and density (Strauss, 1987).
- Analysis of data aims to discover the dominant themes and later generate a conceptual framework which underpins the emerging theory (Glaser and Strauss, 1967).

In a well-constructed grounded theory there are four essential criteria for appraising the applicability of a theory to a phenomenon:

1. fit
2. understanding
3. generality
4. control (Glaser and Strauss, 1967).

The researcher aims at capturing all of the variations in the phenomenon under study and looking at all of the conditions under which the phenomenon occurs, as well as any conditions under which it changes. Data collection, examination, coding, categorising, conceptualising and writing all occur at the same time (Glaser and Strauss, 1967). Hypotheses and theories materialise from the data set while the data collection is proceeding and concurrently with data analysis.

THE PROCESS

When the group meetings began, the men's partners were in the second trimester of pregnancy. The men attended a series of five meetings and subsequent individual interviews. Additional data and insights were gained by the researcher (Donovan) and the research assistant (England) attending other antenatal classes with men and women present. The research data consisted of

- transcripts of tape-recorded interviews,
- group discussions,
- observations and

- field notes made by the researcher (Donovan) and co-leader (Ramsay) following each of the group's sessions.

The aim was to systematically develop a substantive grounded theory which was drawn from the experiences of the men during this transitional period in their lives. This chapter discusses the relationship of existing literature with the five theoretical constructs which emerged from the data collected from the group. These five theoretical constructs were:

1. ambivalence in the early stages of pregnancy,
2. relationship with baby not real,
3. how should I be as a father?
4. coping with the changing roles and lifestyle, and
5. disequilibrium in the relationship with the female partner.

This last construct emerged as the basic social process or core category. Emotional turmoil and anxiety in the men contributed to the mismatch in male and female expectations of the relationship. Ambivalence in the early stages of pregnancy and anxiety about producing a normal baby contributed to the men's feeling of separateness from the growing foetus. The women focused increasingly on the baby growing within and the women's emotions centred on their own feelings as the pregnancy progressed. The relationship between the two expectant partners was changing constantly and the men felt remote from their partner as well as being anxious and confused. The men wondered if their lives would ever return to normal.

The findings of this and later research (Barclay and Donovan, 1995) suggested that current antenatal classes did not meet the needs of the male partner (Barclay et al., 1995).

RELATIONSHIP OF THE THEORETICAL SCHEMA TO EXISTING LITERATURE

1. Ambivalence in the early stages of pregnancy

The findings in this study indicate that, for the group, the transition through pregnancy to parenthood was a process of continual change and uncertainty.

In the beginning stages of pregnancy most men in the group were ambivalent about the event and wondered whether they really wanted to have children. Some said that there were already too many children in the world. The initial ambivalence was combined with feelings of being out of touch with what was going on, while their female partners felt great excitement. Anxiety was displayed in many group sessions. Most of the men were worried about whether their baby would be normal.

These findings are congruent with the literature and are supported by Hobbs and Cole (1976), Meyerowitz and Feldman (1966) and Russell (1974). LeMasters (1957) also highlighted the myth of parenthood as a factor which contributed to the difficulty of adjustment. His conclusion was that the transition to parenthood was a crisis period, however, more recent studies have described it as a normative transition (Combrinck-Graham, 1985; May, 1982). May's work (1982) discusses the ambivalence men experience, particularly during the

> announcement phase — the period during which the pregnancy was first suspected and then confirmed (May, 1982:339).

Bittman and Zalk (1987) confirm the finding of ambivalence of men in early pregnancy. May (1982) highlights the fact that men feel 'uprooted' by the news and may even 'withdraw' temporarily from the situation to 'take care of himself'. Colman and Colman (1971:120), state that

> some pregnancies will instantly bring joy, others anxiety.

Lederman (1984:30) believes that if ambivalence is maintained in the third trimester this is an indication of 'unresolved conflicts'. Lederman also suggests that high ambivalence may indicate low acceptance of the pregnancy, which agrees with some of the views of our participants about their own ambivalence.

Jordan (1990) believes that societal beliefs about gender roles help to support the view that men are the helpers and supporters of the woman during pregnancy, thus contributing to men's feelings of ambivalence. It is reported by Bittman and Zalk (1978:51) that 'there is universal fear of birth defects', and that men become anxious about their own ability and future competence as fathers. May (1982) expands on this view and states that it is thought that men are compelled to confront their future life and resources as they progress through the pregnancy, which, for most men, produces anxiety.

2. Relationship with baby unreal

In the second trimester of pregnancy men have little evidence of the pregnancy, and May (1982) states that it is characteristic of the man to distance himself emotionally because he feels strongly that the baby is not yet real. May (1982) further comments that when men did not feel any connection with the baby they often reacted to the situation by withdrawing further from their partner. May (1982) thought that the fathers' ambivalence resolution was necessary before identification with the foetus and, subsequently, preparation for the labor, delivery and beginning of the parenting role could occur.

The expressions voiced in our group when the partners were before the twenty-fifth week of pregnancy affirmed the validity of May's findings:

- *Nothing has happened yet.*
- *No big deal.*
- *I don't all of a sudden feel a great responsibility or connection with the unborn baby as yet.*
- *What's the fuss about?*

Individual members of the group said in the interviews after the baby was born that they wished at that time, when they had distanced themselves from their partner, that their partner had shown concern, by asking about their own needs, but they were not asked.

Bittman and Zalk (1978) also agree with the view of our group that society in general reinforces the feeling that the father is the outsider in this new relationship and is expected to take on the role of financial supporter and supporter of the woman. This is emphasised in the way antenatal classes are conducted (Bittman and Zalk, 1978). Some of the men in our group agreed that the baby would not feel real to them until they met face to face at the birth.

3. How should I be as a father during pregnancy?

Most of the men in our group thought their partners wanted them to be involved in preparing for the new baby, but there was disagreement about how this would be achieved. They spoke at length around their own intergenerational experiences and about how they wanted to be different from their own parents but they had no role models.

Increased ambiguity in who does what during pregnancy has led to increased confusion in the household (Entwisle and Doering, 1981). Certainly, the man gets the message from society that 'thou shalt take care of the little woman' (Bittman and Zalk, 1978) and sometimes this gets in the way while he is trying to sort out just 'who he is in relation to his new family' (Bittman and Zalk, 1978:410). In some cases the female partner is resistant to her male partner being involved in household tasks and being interested in the foetus. If the man wants to be involved, there can sometimes be considerable unrest and confusion (Entwisle and Doering, 1981). Many writers agree that pregnancy invokes reminders of childhood — how one was parented, loss, and other intergenerational experiences (Combrinck-Graham, 1985; Bittman and Zalk, 1978). The memories are often painful; for example, emotions of what it was like to be fathered as a child living in poverty may stir up the compelling need to overprovide now (Bittman and Zalk, 1978; Colman and Colman, 1971). For the first-time father, pregnancy is the time 'to incorporate father into your self-image' and 'is a man's time to develop this role, to give shape to this new image' (Bittman and Zalk, 1978:166). This is supported by Colman and Colman (1971) and clearly links into the theoretical construct, 'how should I be as a father?'

Herzog (1982) thought that men often returned to their father to sort out who and how they wanted to be in their own new image. In our study it was difficult for the men who, referring to their 'traditional fathers', found marked differences from what is expected today. This resulted in confusion and disequilibrium. Combrinck-Graham (1985:145) also agrees with the view and adds that

> the first child's birth usually effects a generational change, everyone moves up a generation. Along with this change comes increased reflection on one's relationships with other generations. Becoming a parent produces more intense reflection on parenting, and these forces often result in a renewal of transgenerational inquiries and associations. There is a change in the composition of the nuclear family when a new person is added and he (sic) believes there is a greater demand for emotional intimacy and availability.

Osofsky (1982:227) states that

> considerable disequilibrium and crisis can herald the beginning of a new growth phase. The conflicts that have been observed in expectant and new fathers appear to be universal. Under optimal circumstances, expectant and new fatherhood would appear to offer the man an opportunity for better resolution of past conflicts and an enhancement of the maturational process. In becoming a parent, reworking the relationship with his partner, and in establishing an interaction with their child, the man has the opportunity — albeit with pain — for greater fulfilment of age-appropriate tasks and enjoyments

This comment links firmly with the findings of our study.

The established literature reports that men traditionally revert to more 'instrumental' role arrangements (i.e. 'doing tasks') during pregnancy and after the birth of the baby (Cowan et al., 1985) and that they also become more 'traditional' in their role (Lamb, 1986). These ideas were clearly evident in our group, as most of the men were mainly concerned with the finances of the family and their own role in the preparation of the house for the forthcoming infant. They came up with the idea that they tended to revert to their own upbringing, which was thought to be traditional. These concerns are also documented by Feldman and Nash (1989) and Hanson and Bozett (1985). In our group some men had increased their working commitment as they were concerned about their ability as providers. According to Bittman and Zalk (1978) this is a well-known concern of expectant fathers.

For those men in our study who wanted to be different from their traditional fathers much confusion arose as they tried to work out their new role, given that they had no established role model. Colman and Colman (1971:99) state that

> our culture simply does not provide meaningful or satisfying roles that will help fathers feel important and expectant.

Even though most of the men in our group attended the antenatal classes they were not sure which was a different role from their own fathers or what their role was. Belsky et al. (1983) and Feldman and Nash (1984) wrote of similar findings — men discussed their own loss of personal hobbies, time to go on overseas trips, and time spent with their partners. Belsky, Lang and Huston (1986:517) found that the more the division of labor changed toward traditionalism, the greater the decline in wives' evaluations of the positive aspects of marriage. Anxiety emerged from the data analysis as a recurring theme in our group and it is frequently reported in the literature (Hanson and Bozett, 1985; Osofsky, 1982).

4. Coping with changing roles and lifestyle

Traditionally fathers have been portrayed as uninvolved in childbirth and childrearing, confined to their role as the family breadwinner and seen to be only the financial provider. The men in our study, most of whom had come from a model of traditional upbringing, were struggling to find the relevance of the traditional role in their own relationship. As well, they were concerned with being the breadwinner and having to cope financially on one salary. At the same time they were dealing with their partner's expectations of them in household matters. Traditionally fathers have not been seen as active participants in the rearing of their children so our men were struggling with this new expectation. Technological, economic and ideological changes in society are redefining what the father is to be but the men in our group tended to look to their own fathers as a role model even though the men realised that this had limited application in today's environment. There was a struggle to deal with changes in lifestyle and the confusing role of father in a changed society.

The transition to parenthood appears to mark the preparation time for a new role as a father. Burr's (1972) role transition theory offers a theoretical framework which links in with this theme identified in our study. He discusses factors such as:

- the clarity of behaviours that make up the role;
- the process involved in learning norms, values and attitudes of the role;
- the amount of help or hindrance the role contributes to reaching personal goals;
- the amount of perceived stress related to complying with expectations of a role; and
- the number and social significance of the changes to be made in a person's life by the new role.

5. Relationship disequilibrium with female partner

Our men said that their relationships were in a state of constant change and turmoil, and that they tried to respond at the time in ways that seemed meaningful to themselves and their family situation. They also reported that emotions were more intense during this time. This was also a finding of

Colman and Colman (1971). Misinterpretation of these intense emotions in turn led to distancing between the couple. As well, the necessity to reorganise the household duties and prioritise social and sporting activities while experiencing personal losses and feeling disconnected to the unborn child challenged the men's willingness to be attentive within the relationship. Cowan et al. (1985) agree with the notion that, for the pregnant couple, becoming a family brings with it constant negative change in relation to various aspects of their mutual lives and their satisfaction as a couple. The major source of dissatisfaction reported in the group was reduction in marital satisfaction due to raised friction and conflict in their relationship. These findings were confirmed in the follow-up interviews with the individual members of our group.

Another cause of disequilibrium was the jealousy that some of the men in the group felt. They said that they envied the developing relationship their partner had with the unborn baby. Their partner's increasing focus and attention towards the unborn child created a sense of rivalry and anxiety within the male. This alienated the men from their relationship. The rivalry was exacerbated because some men felt that their partner should be taking the time to consider their needs as well. This finding was reiterated in the follow-up interviews as being one aspect with which individuals found it very difficult to cope. Some men felt that they would have liked to have been reassured by their partner that their needs would be met as they normally were after the baby was born. A cause of great concern was not knowing whether the relationship was going to continue as it had been before the feeling of being mismatched or in relationship disequilibrium. Anderson (1984) mentions how jealousy in the expectant man can be experienced either in the form of overidentification with his partner, when he experiences pregnancy physically, or by denying the pregnancy while feeling jealous of his partner and the unborn foetus. This is also supported by Bittman and Zalk (1987), Entwisle and Doering (1981), Shapiro (1987) and Swanson (1980) who highlight the enormous resentment which builds up in many men when their partner, while demanding to be looked after in extra ways, forgets — because they are pregnant — to be concerned or understanding of their male partner's needs. 'Although it is important for the expectant woman to turn inwards and begin bonding with the life forming within her body' (Shapiro, 1987), it is not surprising that so many men feel left out of the relationship. Condon (1987) also found in his sample of couples that the men experienced more 'marital insecurity' than their female partner, because they were so worried and feared that their partner would be closer to the newborn baby than to them. Although the men in our group were busy with activities such as painting the baby's room they did not feel that their wishes were considered.

A further factor causing discomposure was the changing body shape of the woman as a result of the pregnancy. In some cases this was seen by the men in the group as beautiful, but for others it created a sense of guilt because they felt that they had been responsible for making their partner so uncomfortable. This was discussed again at length in the follow-up interviews when the men reported that the combination of morning sickness and excessive tiredness led to a reduction or lessened urge to make love. This was also supported by

Bittman and Zalk (1978) and May (1987). At the same time, the female partner tended to look for extra support and nurturing (Entwisle and Doering, 1981) and many of the men seemed unable to show support and nurturing apart from sex. In many instances in our study it was found that the female partner became more dependent on the male partner and did not consider males had any needs. Colman and Colman (1971) also found that females were unable to understand what their partners were experiencing despite their increased dependence. Colman and Colman suggested that the couple in a partnership should develop a

> new alliance, an agreement to be sensitive to one another's needs, to communicate what is needed now from one another, to share experiences to help the other cope with the unfamiliar and frightening (Colman and Colman, 1971:118).

This is also supported by Shapiro (1987).

Some of our men knew that it was necessary to talk to their partners about the changes within their sexual relationship, realising that there was a mismatch in desire and need. As previously stated, most felt that their partners were not in tune nor acknowledging the male partner's needs but were tending to focus in on the growing foetus and the new relationship that was forming. The men felt excluded from this new relationship — the baby was not real to them. This finding has also been supported by Jordan (1990), Lederman (1984) and Shapiro (1987). What tended to happen was that the men were not used to the changes and were unable to talk openly about their needs which often led to the female partner thinking that they were being rejected by the male. Bittman and Zalk (1978) recommend that couples should talk about their feelings.

One theme that was explored in the group was the notion that female partners were more emotional during pregnancy and that they were demanding more emotional support but their communication signals were 'hard to read'. Some of the men said that their female partners were unclear about their needs which made it more difficult for the male partner to respond immediately and appropriately and often they did nothing. In some instances, they did not respond to their partner intentionally because they were feeling very frustrated and anxious which resulted in a 'mismatch of emotional need'. Most of the men agreed that they tended to 'get wound up, but continue on' as if nothing had changed, despite receiving confusing signals from their partner. They agreed that often their way of responding to the demands of the female partner was by

- doing more,
- tending to tasks like working at house repairs, and
- not taking time out to find out what was really occurring emotionally with their female partner.

Most of the men observed what was going on from the sidelines; they felt like an outsider while the female became absorbed in the growing baby. Lederman

(1984:15) says that the pregnant woman is in

> the preparatory process for creation (which) almost always involves periods of withdrawal, brooding introspection and intensified sensibility, and it is close to the indescribable world of the unconscious, for this is an inner process. The creating person is, therefore, essentially alone — despite all the encouragement and adulation she might receive — and what she does necessarily has some degree of stress and tension. She works for and waits for the work of art to take on a life of its own and at a certain moment puts it forth for the world to see. The creative act also requires that the creating person separate herself from her production; and, again, in terms of both figures in the analogy, mother and child, the creating person feels a sense of accomplishment.

The men wished their partner would say what they actually wanted but they seemed unable to. This links in with the work of Swanson (1980) and Shapiro (1987) who found, in some instances, that some men had extramarital affairs at this time with women they felt they could talk to because communication with their pregnant partners was so confusing and the men felt their own needs were not being considered at all. The men in our group commented that if they were not communicating well within the relationship then this would naturally feed into their sexuality. Perkins (1984) and May (1987:62) also believe that

> most adults see their marital relationship as central to their lives and as a major source of satisfaction.

Masturbation as a normal outlet is discussed by Bittman and Zalk (1978) who found that men tended to masturbate more often in the first and third trimesters of pregnancy. Most of the men in our group confirmed in the individual interviews that they masturbated, especially in the third trimester of the pregnancy.

THE MODEL

The model devised as a result of our research is illustrated in Figure 11.1 (see opposite page)

Figure 11.1 From category to core category through theoretical constucts using grounded theory

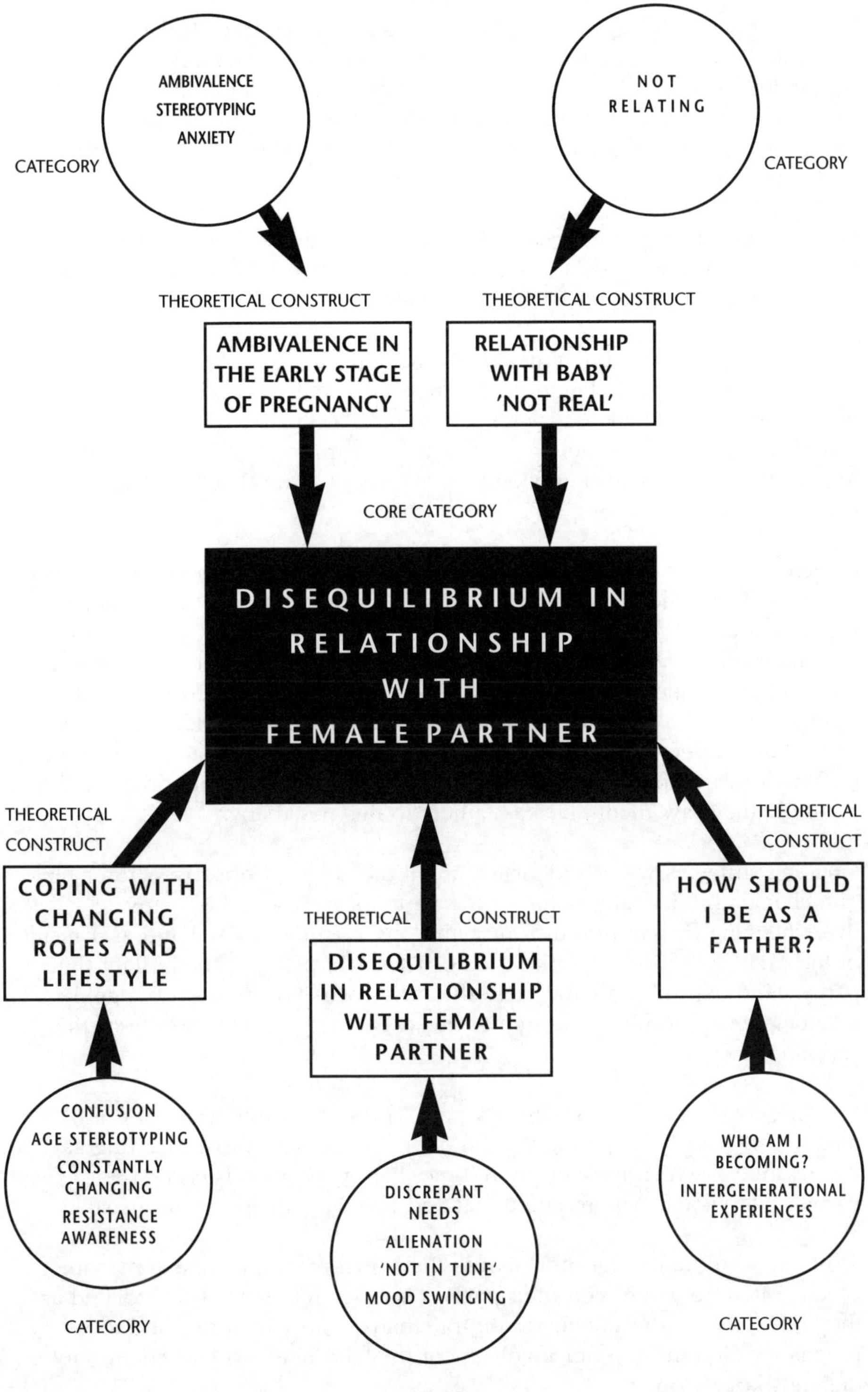

CONCLUSION

Many men who are in transition to fatherhood today face the dilemma of having a father who was brought up in the traditional role. Today's men, therefore, have no role model exhibiting the characteristics desired or demanded of them. Understanding the changing roles and experiences of men within their pregnant partnership needs to be held foremost in the minds of clinicians who are interacting with men and helping them to solve problems.

Being part of a pregnancy raises many issues for men. These include personal thoughts about having children and what this means within a partnership, and thoughts about losses of time and friendships.

Experiences such as a previous miscarriage or other loss, for example stillbirth, were raised at length in this research until those men in our group who were affected had dealt with it to their own satisfaction. It was something the men had never spoken about or processed for themselves before. In the follow-up interviews the men said again that they had been very anxious about having an abnormal baby.

It seems that only through being asked specific questions, in an environment in which their needs were of concern, when they were apart from their female partner, did the men feel comfortable about revealing and dealing with their inner concerns. Initially, they had found it difficult to relate to the unborn baby, which was quite unreal to them. They struggled with their changing role and lifestyle and with how they could incorporate their own and others' expectations into these roles. They reflected on how they were parented, related present experiences and ideals and thought about the future and how they saw themselves as fathers to this new baby.

Ongoing struggles were evident within all the couples' primary partnerships. The changing, uncertain nature of the partnership resulted in many overwhelming feelings, both from within the men themselves and as a result of their partner's more emotional state. The male participants thought their partner and the unborn baby were the main focus for attention by family members, health professionals and others. The male was seen only as the support person.

Society's expectations also played a part. The participants were all doing men's work, busily preparing for the baby with great gusto and acting as breadwinners, which took up more time than was appreciated by their partner, who wanted more emotional and intimate attention than usual.

Most expectant fathers do not discuss their own emotional reactions with others, often not even with their partner, so they feel somewhat isolated as they make these adjustments during pregnancy. How men respond to pregnancy, and the level of involvement they are likely to find comfortable, depends largely on

- their personality,
- their sex role expectations,
- their previous experiences with hospital and physical pain, and
- whether the pregnancy was planned and desired.

Current trends and activities in antenatal education in some institutions aim to include the male partner but still have a long way to go towards offering services that focus on the dyad specifically and then on the female and the male individually. Most postnatal services focus entirely on the mother and baby, despite calling themselves family-centred services.

As was seen in our study, the evolution of the fathering role can be viewed from a developmental framework. The transition to parenthood takes men and women from a known life phase to an unknown phase. The experience encompasses many challenging situations which present as disequilibrium in the couple's relationship.

References

Anderson I (1984): Transition to parenthood research. *Journal of Psychometric Obstetrics and Gynaecology* 3: 3–16.

Barclay L and Donovan J (1994): The preparation for parenting — experiences of men in classes, paper presented at 'Families our Future — Preconception to Parenthood', Fourth Biennial Conference of the National Association of Childbirth Educators. Canberra. September.

Barclay L, Donovan J and Genovese A (1996): Men's experiences during their partner's first pregnancy: A grounded theory analysis. *Australian Journal of Advanced Nursing* 13 3: 12–24.

Belsky J, Spanier GB and Rovine M (1983): Stability and change in marriage across the transition to parenthood. *Journal of Marriage and the Family* 45: 567–77.

Belsky J, Lang M and Huston TL (1986): Sex typing and division of labor as determinants of marital change across the transition to parenthood. *Journal of Personality and Social Psychology* 50 3: 517–22.

Bittman S and Zalk SR (1987): *Expectant Fathers*. New York: Hawthorn Books.

Burr WR 1972: Role transition: A reformulation of theory. *Journal of Marriage and the Family* 34: 407–16.

Colman A and Colman L (1971): *Pregnancy: The Psychological Experience*. New York: Herder and Herder.

Combrinck-Graham L (1985): A developmental model for family systems. *Family Process* 24 2: 139–50.

Condon J (1987): Psychological and physical symptoms during pregnancy: A comparison of male and female expectant parents. *Journal of Reproductive and Infant Psychology* 5: 207–19.

Cowan CP, Cowan PA, Herning G, Garrett E, Coysh WS, Curtis Bates HJ and Boles AJ (1985): Transitions to parenthood: His, hers and theirs. *Journal of Family Issues* 6: 451–81.

Donovan J (1994): Men's social, emotional and sexual responses to their partner's pregnancy. Master of Science thesis, Flinders University, South Australia.

Donovan J (1995): The process of analysis during a grounded theory study of men during their partners' pregnancies. *Journal of Advanced Nursing* 21: 708–15.

Entwisle DR and Doering SG (1981): *The First Birth: A Family Turning Point?* Baltimore and London: Johns Hopkins University Press.

Feldman SS and Nash SC (1984): The transition from pregnancy to parenthood: Impact of the firstborn child on men and women. *Sex Roles* 111–2: 61–78.

Glaser BG and Strauss AL (1967): *The Discovery of Grounded Theory: Strategies for Qualitative Research*. New York: Aldine.

Hanson SMH and Bozett FW (eds) (1985): *Dimensions of Fatherhood*. California: Sage.

Herzog JM (1982): Patterns of Expectant Fatherhood: A Study of the Fathers of a Group of Premature Infants. In: Cath SH, Gurwitt AR and Ross JM (eds): *Father and Child*. Boston: Little Brown.

Hobbs DF and Cole SP (1976): Transition to parenthood: A decade replication. *Journal of Marriage and the Family* 38: 723–32.

Jordan PL (1990): Laboring for relevance: Expectant and new fatherhood. *Nursing Research* 39 1: 11–16.

Lamb ME (1986): The Changing Roles of Father. In Lamb ME (ed.): *The Father's Role: Applied Perspectives*. New York: Wiley.

LeMasters EE (1957): Parenthood as crisis. *Marriage and Family Living* 19: 322–355.

Lederman RP (1984): *Psychosocial Adaption in Pregnancy*. Englewood Cliffs, New Jersey: Prentice Hall.

May KA (1982): Three phases of father involvement in pregnancy. *Nursing Research* 31: 337–42.

May KA (1987): Men's sexuality during the childbearing year: Implications of recent research findings. *Holistic Nursing Practice* 1 4: 60–66.

Meyerowitz JH and Feldman H (1966): Transition to parenthood. *Psychiatric Research Report*. 20: 78–84.

Osofsky H 1982: Expectant and new fatherhood as a developmental crisis. *Bulletin of the Menninger Clinic* 46 3: 209–30.

Perkins RP (1984): Sexuality during pregnancy. *Clinical Obstetrics and Gynaecology* 27 3: 706–16.

Russell CS (1974): Transition to parenthood: Problems and gratification. *Journal of Marriage and the Family* 36: 294–302.

Shapiro JL (1987): *When Men Are Pregnant — Needs and Concerns of Expectant Fathers*. California: Impact Publishers.

Strauss AL (1987): *Qualitative Analysis for Social Scientists*. New York: University Press.

Swanson J (1980): The marital sexual relationship during pregnancy. *Journal of Obstetric, Gynaecology and Neonatal Nursing* 9 5: 267–70.

Terry DJ (1991): Stress, coping and adaption to new parenthood. *Journal of Social and Personal Relationships* 8: 527–47.

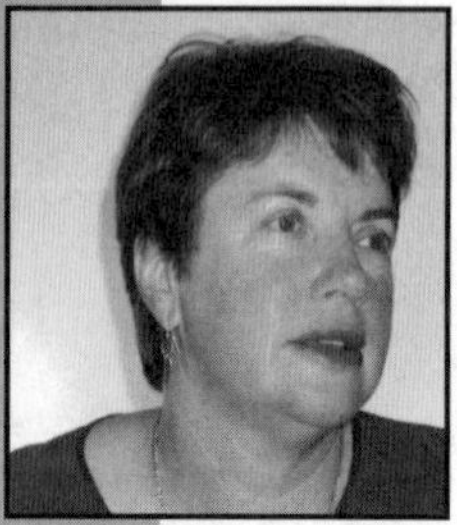

JENNY DONOVAN

Registered Nurse, Registered Midwife, Certificate of Maternal and Child Health, Bachelor of Nursing, Master of Science (Primary Health Care), Fellow of the Royal College of Nursing, Australia

Jenny Donovan wrote this of herself and this chapter:

I am working as a lecturer in nursing at The Flinders University of South Australia while completing a PhD part-time at RMIT University in Melbourne. My most recent experience was as the Manager of Family and Children's Services at the Brimbank Community Health Service in the Western suburbs of Melbourne, now named ISIS Primary Care. My current project is about the experiences of men and women as they prepare for another baby, given a previous experience of treated postnatal depression in the female partner. My research and teaching interests focus on the transition to parenthood for men and women (including adolescents), with a particular focus on parenting issues. At present I am also involved in a large research team looking at men's role in parenting. I have always lived in a blended family and understand the challenges and demands required. My love of animals and music keep me sane!

Special thanks to the Post and Antenatal Association (PaNDa) of Victoria for their support and encouragement, and also to the participants in the project, who shared their stories with me.

Chapter Twelve

'Walking on eggshells': postnatal depression and subsequent parenting for men

INTRODUCTION

Much has been written concerning the mental health effects of postnatal depression for women, but the effect on male partners has not previously been explored. This chapter highlights the need to develop a body of knowledge about men's health that goes beyond the mainstream concerns of physical wellbeing.

The chapter begins by highlighting the facts that:

- mental illness is grossly underrecognised in our community;
- health services operating under direction of current policy initiatives do not adequately meet the needs of those suffering mental health problems; and
- contemporary gender roles generate unnecessary stresses that can contribute to mental health problems.

This contextualisation is essential to gain a heightened appreciation of the fact that, for both sexes, the stresses developing in connection with pregnancy and parenthood may be superimposed on pre-existing life stressors that are not insignificant.

MENTAL HEALTH IN AUSTRALIA

Approximately 20 per cent of the Australian population will suffer some kind of mental health problem or mental disorder in a year (Raphael, 1993). A study by Rey (1992) revealed that about one in five mental illnesses begin in early adolescence and early adulthood; however, mental health services in Australia deal mainly with middle-aged or elderly adults, leaving adolescents and young adults floundering (Kosky and Hardy, 1992).

In Rey's study 29 per cent of the men and 31 per cent of the women had suffered a mental disorder in the previous year, with men having a higher incidence of alcohol abuse, drug abuse and antisocial personality and women a higher incidence of depressive and anxiety disorders.

> In adulthood, men experience more alcohol and drug abuse and antisocial behaviour, while women experience more anxiety, depression and eating disorders (Jorm, 1995:vi).

It is also well known that males are more likely to commit suicide than females and that those who suffer from a mental disorder are at a greater risk (Goldney, 1995). The literature also suggests that more attention needs to be given to solving the problem of suicide in men; current strategies are more effective in assisting suicidal women than men (Lester, 1995).

An example of how men and women react differently to emotional pain and stress has been illustrated by the Family and Child Health Study. This longitudinal study of bereaved parents and their matched non-bereaved controls (Boyle, 1994) found that men and women respond differently to the same events, and that the way this response is measured determines which group is perceived to have the highest rate of mental disorders.

Schoenborn and Horm (1993) highlighted the fact that negative mood, nicotine dependence and alcohol abuse more often coexist in men than in women, and signal mental disorder. It is also known that men with more serious states of mental disorder may find themselves being dealt with by other agencies, for example the criminal justice system, rather than by psychiatric services (Najman, 1995:9). Men have had to accept a decrease in their power and control in marriage and this can create role changes and demands on men which are likely to affect their mental health. Najman talks about mental disorder as created by the prevalent social structures. Najman (1995:17-18) notes that:

- increasing rates of unemployment and particularly long-term unemployment [are] disproportionately impacting on men. There are many mental and physical health consequences of these patterns of unemployment;
- changes within the family [are] leading to the erosion of male patriarchy and requiring men to give up some of their power and dominance;
- changes in family life [are] such that marriage is a more flexible institution, with increasing proportions of the population experiencing marital changes. Such changes are associated with a wide range of marital and physical health problems; and
- [there is] an apparent increase in the rate at which children are abandoned by parents, with a disproportionate number of these being boys.

Research demonstrates that general practitioners treat only about 40 per cent of those who present with a mental disorder (Andrews, 1991). The National Mental Health Policy and Plan (DHHCS, 1992) highlights general practitioners' important role in recognising and treating mental conditions while recognising the need for improvement (Paykel and Priest, 1992) as well as diagnostic precision and management (Ormel et al., 1990). There is also a need to understand the stigma surrounding mental illness and patients' feelings of discomfort about being referred to psychiatrists and other relevant mental health professionals (Phongsavan et al., 1995).

Other areas worthy of discussion are men's exposure to war and the significance of unemployment in relation to the traditional notion of masculine identity (the breadwinner). Studies by Faustman and White (1989) and Kulka et al. (1990) demonstrate an association of high rates of concurrent psychiatric disorders (e.g. mood disorders, substance-use disorders and other anxiety disorders) with war zone-related post-traumatic stress disorder. A more recent study strengthens the view that war zone-related post-traumatic stress disorder is associated with high rates of psychiatric comorbidity (Orsillo et al., 1995) although O'Toole et al. (1995:60) recognise that:

> the diagnosis of the disorder and its differentiation from other disorders are not always easily accomplished.

Increasingly research is demonstrating that stresses experienced in emergency and other organisational services (ambulance, police, firefighters, shiftworkers and others) may lead to mental health problems, particularly when workers do not acknowledge their experiences (Meldrum and Raphael, 1995).

Barnett et al. (1992) and Repetti (1989) examined the relationship between men's multiple roles and men's psychological distress. Barnett and Marshall (1992) found that the relationship between job stress and psychological distress was exacerbated among men who had troubled relationships with their partners. According to Campbell et al. (1976), the most powerful predictor of an individual's quality of life is that person's reported quality of relationship with his/her partner.

WORK AND FAMILY

Having established the tensions that exist in Australian society regarding mental health it is appropriate at this point to consider the additional stresses that can develop in connection with pregnancy and parenthood for both sexes. Increasingly the men's movement encourages men to be involved more actively in the care of their children (Hanson and Bozett, 1986). However, heavy competition, the changing role of men and women and the lower levels of family stability have brought careers and the home into potential conflict (Friedman et al., 1997:6). Increasingly employers are aware of the importance to business success of creating an environment that values diversity and encourages a balance between work and family responsibilities; the challenge for larger corporations is to coordinate these strategies across a diverse range of businesses (Guazzarotto, 1997:8). Workplaces that fail to recognise the changes that are occurring will suffer in the long run as men and women struggle to find their places in society. The workplace needs to be aware of major changes which occur in the family life cycle, for instance, pregnancy.

THE PREGNANT COUPLE

Pregnancy, as a major transitional period in adulthood, presents many challenges and stresses for the pregnant couple (Campbell and Field, 1989) and poses challenges to the family life cycle (Combrinck-Graham, 1985) and to all components of relationship dynamics (Tomlinson et al., 1990). Osofsky (1982:226) states that expectant and new fatherhood creates a

> developmental opportunity for maturation and new growth.

According to Feldman and Nash (1984:62)

> one of the most dramatic transitions in the family life cycle, experienced by more than 80 per cent of all adults, occurs between the stages of expectancy and parenthood.

THE MAN DURING PREGNANCY

Bothamley (1990) stresses that social and emotional changes are not uniquely female and are known to occur in the male during the course of his partner's pregnancy. Research undertaken more than a decade ago demonstrated that an expectant father experiences developmental processes, stresses and adjustment behaviours that are as individual and diverse as those associated with pregnancy in a woman (May, 1982a).

May (1982c) states that men may undergo changes in their emotional and behavioural responses to pregnancy over time, beginning with the emergence and resolution of emotional worries about expectant fatherhood and moving later in pregnancy toward highlighting their role in pregnancy and birth and their prospective roles as fathers. May also found that, during their partner's pregnancy, men had three separate styles of involvement ranging from detachment to active involvement. May described these styles as:

- observer style;
- expressive style; and
- instrumental style.

From the data collected in his work, May (1982c) identified three phases in men's changing perceptions of pregnancy:

- the announcement;

- the moratorium; and
- the focusing.

May (1982a) also found four factors which contributed to men's readiness for fatherhood and emotional involvement:

- relative financial security;
- an intention to become a parent;
- a sense of conclusion to the childless period of the marital relationship; and
- perceived stability in the marital relationship.

For those men for whom the pregnancy had come too soon, the four factors were not in place, which influenced the men's propensity to support the woman in pregnancy and during and after labour. Men who seemed disappointed by, detached from or ambivalent about the pregnancy might experience disruption in the primary relationship (May, 1982a). Health professionals coming into contact with these men might label them as indifferent or unsupportive men.

Two authors, Jordan (1990) and Swanson (1980), depict pregnancy as essentially a time of identity transition, when men are 'labouring for relevance' (Jordan, 1990:12) and struggling for recognition as a parent. Men's need for companionship and support during pregnancy has been covered already in chapter 11 of this book. Many other studies which focus on men during pregnancy cover areas such as:

- emotional response linked to health status (Clinton, 1986:294);
- mismatched sexual interest levels (Barclay et al., 1994);
- social and emotional experiences (Donovan, 1994, 1995);
- general stress (Clinton, 1986:294);
- jealousy of their partners (McNall, 1976);
- role change (Russell, 1983);
- social support (Brown 1986);
- couvade (especially in ethnic minorities) (Drake et al., 1988); and
- family systems development (Combrinck-Graham, 1985).

Traditionally health professionals and researchers have focused on women's physical changes and emotions (Imle, 1990) with specific emphasis on the preparation for labour. Expectant fathers are expected by society in general, health professionals and their female partners, to be present at the delivery (Jordan, 1990; Bothamley, 1990) and to anticipate their partner's needs (Longobucco and Freston, 1989) despite often being unprepared for it

(Bothamley, 1990). May (1982b:319) supports the notion that many clinicians and childbirth educators

> hold an unrealistic expectation of fathers, as though there is an 'ideal' expectant father.

Current practice in obstetric and midwifery perpetuates these ideas. Couples are encouraged to attend antenatal classes in the third trimester of pregnancy. Given the magnitude of social, emotional and sexual changes experienced by most pregnant couples far earlier in the pregnancy (Barclay et al., 1994), antenatal classes held in the last trimester appear to be too late to address the changes that occur in the relationship between partners. The changing relationship of couples during pregnancy would seem to provide a significant opportunity during this transitional period for increased maturation and growth for the male (Osofsky, 1982). However, there is a dearth of research which examines men's experiences and their responses during pregnancy (Bothamley, 1990; Imle, 1990; Jordan, 1990). The developmental changes experienced by men during pregnancy, if not recognised and dealt with in the antenatal period, may lead to increased stress and impairment of psychological function (Campbell, 1989). It appears likely that these changes may have ramifications for the pregnant couple's relationship.

POSTNATAL DEPRESSION

Just how much of the tension outlined above plays a role in the incidence and severity of postnatal depression is not known but researchers are beginning to examine men's experiences of their partner's postnatal depression. The questions yet to be answered are:

- Do men understand the causes, signs and symptoms of postnatal depression?
- What is their appreciation and understanding of mental health problems?
- What part does their own mental health or family background play in these situations?
- Do men have any resources to help them support their partner and, as a result, themselves?

The first description of postnatal mental illness in women dates back to Hippocrates in the fourth century BC (Holden, 1991:211). In 1858, in his *Traite de la Folie des Femmes Enceintes,* Marce investigated 310 examples of mental illness in women associated with childbearing (Rickel, 1984). Initial literature focuses on psychotic reactions (Seager, 1960) with later interest focusing on other possible causes attributed to postpartum disturbance. It was not until the late 1960s that more

> experimental work on postpartum disturbance began appearing (Rickel, 1984:198).

All of the work conducted at this time focused on the female partner.

Australian and international figures quoting the incidence of postnatal depression vary from 10 to 15 per cent in all births (Holden et al., 1989). Postpartum depression is more serious and longer lasting than the transitory depression and crying spells after childbirth, which occur in about 60 per cent of women (Stein, 1984) and are commonly referred to as the 'maternity blues'. It is less serious than 'postpartum psychosis' which is characterised by extremely altered perceptions of reality (Kumar and Robson, 1984). Postpartum depression

- may begin within the first weeks after delivery and persist for months, sometimes years (Watson et al., 1984);
- often occurs unrecognised (Gerrard et al., 1993); and
- occurs in all cultures and social classes (Ball, 1986).

Adcock (1993:704) points out that contemporary literature attributes postnatal depression to a variety of reasons which may include a combination of psychological, socioeconomic, biochemical and physical factors. Most research in the area of postnatal depression reveals extensive quantitative designs which focus almost exclusively on the mother or the mother and child dyad (Milgrom, 1994) with little attention being paid to the male partner. Available qualitative literature continues the focus on the woman (Beck, 1992;1993).

According to Lovestone and Kumar (1993) an area requiring investigation is that which describes the experiences for expectant men where there has been postnatal depression diagnosed in their partner in a previous pregnancy. Research in 1995 by Dudley cites the high prevalence of psychological disorders in fathers attending mothercraft services in Sydney (Michael Dudley, personal communication). In a recent study by Brown et al. (1994) women said that they found it difficult to find someone to talk to about their depression and, in particular, did not discuss their fears with their male partners, who were not included in the study. It is not generally known who men talk to about their own or their partner's depression. We know that male psychiatric morbidity is increased when their partner has been admitted to a mother and baby unit (Harvey and McGrath, 1988) and that postnatal depression can have major effects on the couple (Watson et al., 1984) and their sexual relationship (Debrovner and Scrubin, 1985).

Most antenatal and self-help groups continue to focus on the needs and circumstances of the mother and child, with little attention being paid to the male partner. Postnatal depression has been documented as becoming chronic in many mothers (Barnett, 1990) and was described by Dudley in 1995 as being prevalent in the male partner (Michael Dudley, personal communication).

POSTNATAL DEPRESSION AND SUBSEQUENT PREGNANCY

A recent Australian grounded theory study (Donovan, 1996) explored men's previous experiences of postpartum depression while expecting another baby with the same partner. The female partners had been identified and labelled by medical practitioners as having had postnatal depression following the birth of their last child. Interviews were conducted with volunteer men and some of their partners antenatally and postnatally through the transition to the birth of their next child. Analysis of the data using the constant comparative method revealed eight elements in the basic social psychological problem:

1. not knowing what to expect;
2. being uncertain;
3. finding out about postnatal depression;
4. trying to fix it;
5. reaching one's limit;
6. accepting our differences;
7. expecting another baby —watching and waiting; and
8. 'hoping we'd come through it'.

Men described their experiences of postnatal depression as 'walking on eggshells'. During the interviews, the men reflected on and recounted their uninformed and unrealistic expectations about the birth experience and becoming a parent for the first time. They had been unable to sort out their own personal needs given their aim to hold the family together and to continue being the breadwinner. They were all working long hours. Few gained support from their workplace, nor did they feel comfortable about sharing their experiences at work. Consequently, silence pervaded and neither the men nor the women sought help early enough. Confusion reigned between myth and reality, expectations, normal postnatal experiences and the experience of postnatal depression. The postnatal depression was seen as the women's problem. The men said they kept on going on, trying not to say or do too much, supporting their partner but fearing that the family would disintegrate from all the pressure they were experiencing. Most of the men received no help from health professionals but were told that they were the support persons, hence their own feelings, experiences and needs were not acknowledged. Seeing postnatal depression as the woman's illness, thus bringing out feelings of inadequacy in her and placing blame on her, may also hinder the couple from solving their own issues together and hence improving their own communication levels.

THE ROLE OF THE HEALTH PROFESSIONAL

We might well consider how we as health professionals work with families as they progress through normal transitions in the family life cycle. In the course of recruiting for the study described above (Donovan, 1996), lengthy telephone discussions were held with men who turned out not to meet the inclusion criteria but who sought the opportunity to debrief their own experiences of previously living in a relationship with a partner who was labelled as having postnatal depression after their first child. Most of the men had never spoken about their experiences before and all blamed their experiences of postnatal depression for their partnership breakup. They vowed that they would never have any more children as their experiences were so painful. None of the men had received any assistance from the health professionals who had worked with their former female partner. The men were either separated or divorced from their previous partner and were mindful of their own unresolved pasts. Other concerned relatives of men rang in to talk about how their brothers had suffered but had not received any personal or professional assistance. Clearly this is another area for research and for creative service provision for men.

As nurses, we do not fully understand what is occurring between women and men who experience another birth given their previous experiences of postnatal depression. It is obvious that we need more research and resources to assist families' individual needs at this time. Additional training will alert all health professionals who work with families through the transition to parenthood to obtain a comprehensive history from both men and women and to follow all cases thoroughly from the antenatal to the postnatal period, particularly taking note of stories that indicate their journey through life to that point. Listening, for instance, to men's personal previous history of depression or family history of depression, unemployment, and any other mediating factors, could contribute towards offering more effective health care within a social view of health. Other ways to acknowledge the needs of both parents could include:

- providing case management with particular emphasis on service responses that agree with client/family needs;
- offering home visits or industry visits to both men and women;
- running a 24-hour crisis parent line;
- providing support groups for men; and
- holding parenting groups in venues and at times when both parents can attend or be contacted.

In particular these parenting groups might cover issues such as:

- anger management;
- changes which occur in both women and men following the birth of the child;
- knowing where to access local resources (for both men and women);
- time management; and
- learning about how to use active listening techniques in the primary relationship and in a nonjudgmental environment.

We know from previous studies that men and women with emotional problems do not seek help actively for their difficulties nor do they discuss them openly. Men, like women, need to be provided with the opportunity to raise their own concerns through the provision of appropriate, relevant and accessible services across primary, secondary and tertiary levels. (Primary health care seeks to focus the health system's first level of contact on promoting and protecting the health of defined communities and on addressing their health problems at an early stage. To do this, primary health care needs to be a network of basic services provided where people live and work. These services must be available to all. Health care at the primary level is backed up by secondary and tertiary levels which contain more specialised services for problems that cannot be handled at the primary level.) (AHMAC, 1988:3).

Issues raised in Barclay's and Donovan's research highlight the need for consistency and collaboration in antenatal and postnatal education within a primary health care framework. In the studies by Barclay and Donovan (1994), Donovan (1995a) and Barclay et al. (1996) and in the work of Donovan reported in this chapter, the male participants indicated that they knew little about many of the normal changes which occur during pregnancy and following the birth of their infants. This was despite the fact that many had attended antenatal courses. Men in Donovan's 1994 thesis suggested that antenatal classes could be structured always to include time to allow the participants to explore and deal with their own enquiries as well as needing to have structured information.

Programs and home visits provided by community midwives antenatally could link both physically and in content with those provided postnatally by other service providers, such as maternal and child health nurses, to bridge the gap between hospital and community within a primary health care framework and to maintain continuity of care for both the client and the professional caregiver. So often the client's needs become lost in the system when too many professionals become involved in the same family. As well, family support workers under the auspices of maternal and child health services could make contact with families antenatally to assist with the provision of a seamless service. Informing families about the normal stresses and differences experienced jointly and separately by men and women might assist them to more successful negotiation within their relationship when faced with additional crises, for instance when depression is experienced by either partner. Creating an environment in which men can support each other informally in times of need is essential. Other services might include critical incident debriefing for men and women as well as for the staff, for example when an emergency Caesarean section has been performed (Mitchell, 1983).

With an improved continuity-of-care approach, families could be linked into appropriate and accessible primary, secondary and tertiary services where necessary. Further needs assessment research could tap into men's inner resources to find out how these services might be offered.
It appears that the concept of 'listening ear visits' as developed by Holden (1993) could be extended to include men who are not being heard nor acknowledged as individuals in this important transition period. Emergency

phone services could improve their telephone services to reach men throughout the community. It is well known that communication levels are impaired when one or both partners are depressed and nurses are well placed to address this issue given their ability and acceptance within the home. Home visits or phone contact currently offered to women, both antenatally by midwives and postnatally by maternal and child health nurses, could be extended to include the male partner in an endeavour to practice more comprehensive family-centred care.

CONCLUSION

Parenthood is a partnership where an understanding of emotional needs and how best they can be supported is central to achieving a good quality of life for parents and children. This chapter has shown that parenting can be severely affected when the needs of men are neglected during their partner's pregnancy and particularly if the pregnancy is followed by postnatal depression. Postnatal depression is a form of mental illness on which some study has been carried out but there are few studies of its effects on men. Mental illness generally is accorded too little attention in our modern society but it is pleasing to see that some efforts are being made to help those who are having and raising the children who constitute our future.

Acknowledgments

The study has been generously supported by the Royal College of Nursing (Myrtle Ivy Quicke Memorial Scholarship), by The Flinders University School of Nursing University Research Board Grant, by the South Australian Institute of Nursing Research Small Grant; and by The Royal Melbourne Institute of Technology University (APA) Scholarship for two years.

The opinions stated in this work are not necessarily those of the Royal College of Nursing, Australia.

References

Adcock JS (1993): Expectations they cannot meet: Understanding postnatal depression. *Professional Nurse* August: 703–10.

Andrews G (1991): The changing nature of psychiatry. *Australian and New Zealand Journal of Psychiatry* 25: 453–59.

Australian Health Ministers Advisory Council (AHMAC) (1988): *Continuing Education for Primary Health Care in Australia,* Report and recommendations. Canberra: AGPS, pp. i–iii, 1–26.

Australian Health Ministers' Conference (1991): *Mental Health Statement of Rights and Responsibilities.* Canberra: AGPS.

Ball JA (1986): Adaptations to motherhood. *Nursing* 2 21: 623–4.

Barclay L and Donovan J (1994): The preparation for parenting — experiences of men in classes, paper presented at 'Families our Future — Preconception to Parenthood', Fourth Biennial Conference of the National Association of Childbirth Educators. Canberra. September.

Barclay L, Donovan J and Genovese A (1996): Men's experiences during their partner's first pregnancy: A grounded theory analysis. *Australian Journal of Advanced Nursing* 13 3: 12–24.

Barclay L, McDonald P and O'Loughlin JA (1994): Sexuality and pregnancy: An interview study. *Australian New Zealand Journal of Obstetrics and Gynaecology* 34 1: 1–7.

Barnett B (1990): Postnatal depression or failure to thrive mothers. *Modern Medicine of Australia* 3: 64–72.

Barnett RC and Marshall NL (1992): Men's job and partner roles: Spillover effects and psychological distress. *Sex Roles* 27 9–10: 455–72.

Barnett RC, Marshall NL and Pleck JH (1992): Men's multiple roles and their relationship to men's psychological distress. *Journal of Marriage and the Family* 54: 358–67.

Beck CT (1992): The lived experience of postpartum depression: A phenomenological study. *Nursing Research* 41 3: 166–70.

Beck CT (1993): Teetering on the edge: A substantive theory of postpartum depression. *Nursing Research* 42 1: 42–8.

Bothamley J (1990): Are fathers getting a fair deal? *Nursing Times* 86 36: 68–9.

Boyle FM (1994): The mental health impact of stillbirth, neonatal death or SIDS: prevalence and patterns of distress among mothers. PhD thesis. Brisbane: University of Queensland.

Brown MA (1986): Marital support during pregnancy. *Journal of Obstetric, Gynaecology and Neonatal Nursing* 15 6: 475–83.

Brown S, Lumley J, Small R and Astbury J (1994): *Missing — The Experience of Motherhood*. Melbourne: Oxford University Press.

Campbell IE and Field PA (1989): Common psychological concerns experienced by parents during pregnancy. *Canada's Mental Health* 37 1: 2–5.

Campbell A, Converse PE and Rodgers WL (1976): *The Quality of American Life: Perceptions, Evaluations and Satisfaction*. New York: Russell Sage.

Clinton JF (1986): Expectant fathers at risk for couvade. *Nursing Research* 35 5: 290–5.

Combrinck-Graham L (1985): A developmental model for family systems. *Family Process* 24 2: 139–50.

Debrovner CH and Scrubin R (1985): Pregnancy and post partum: II Post partum sexual concerns. *Medical Aspects of Human Sexuality* 19 5, May: 84–90.

Department of Health, Housing and Community Services (DHHCS) (1992): *National Mental Health Policy and Plan*. Canberra: AGPS.

Donovan J (1994): Men's social, emotional and sexual responses to their partner's pregnancy. Master of Science thesis, Flinders University, South Australia.

Donovan J (1995): The process of analysis during a grounded theory study of men during their partners' pregnancies. *Journal of Advanced Nursing* 21: 708–15.

Donovan J (1996): The impact of postnatal depression on the male partner: A study of men in Victoria, paper presented at 'Choice is a Challenge': conference of the National Association of Childbirth Educators, Adelaide. Part of a PhD thesis in progress, Department of Nursing, RMIT University, Melbourne.

Drake ML, Verhulst D and Fawcett J (1988): Physical and psychological symptoms experienced by Canadian women and their husbands during pregnancy and the postpartum. *Journal of Advanced Nursing* 13: 436–40.

Faustman WO and White PA (1989): Diagnostic and psychopharmacological treatment characteristics of 536 patients with post-traumatic stress disorder. *Journal of Nervous and Mental Disease* 171: 585–96.

Feldman SS and Nash SC (1984): The transition from pregnancy to parenthood: Impact of the firstborn child on men and women. *Sex Roles* 11 1–2: 61–78.

Friedman S, Christensen P and DeGroot J (1997): Business must balance more than its books. *Business Review Weekly* 17 March.

Gerrard J, Holden JM, Elliott SA, McKenzie P, McKenzie J and Cox JL (1993): A trainer's perspective of an innovative programme teaching health visitors about the detection, treatment and prevention of postnatal depression. *Journal of Advanced Nursing* 18: 1825–1832.

Goldney RD (1995): Suicide in Men. In: National Health and Medical Research Council (ed.): *Men and Mental Health*. Canberra: AGPS.

Guazzarotto D (1997): Coles Myer Ltd: Managing diversity in a large organisation. *Work & Family* 13: 1–16.

Hanson SMH and Bozett FW (1986): The changing nature of fatherhood: The nurse and social policy. *Journal of Advanced Nursing* 11: 719–27.

Harvey I and McGrath G (1988): Psychiatric morbidity in spouses of women admitted to a mother and baby unit. *British Journal of Psychiatry* 152, April: 506–10.

Holden J, Sagovsky R and Cox JL (1989): Counselling in general practice setting: A controlled study of health visitor intervention in treatment of post natal depression. *British Medical Journal* 298: 223–6.

Holden J (1991): Postnatal depression: Its nature, effects and identification using the Edinburgh Postnatal Depression Scale. *Birth* 18 4: 211–21.

Imle M (1990): Third trimester concerns of expectant parents in transition to parenthood. *Holistic Nursing Practice* 4 3: 11–16.

Jordan PL (1990): Labouring for relevance: Expectant and new fatherhood. *Nursing Research* 39 1: 11–16.

Jorm AF (1995): Executive summary. In: National Health and Medical Research Council (ed.): *Men and Mental Health*. Canberra: AGPS.

Kosky R and Hardy J (1992): Mental health: Is early intervention the key? *The Medical Journal of Australia* 156: 147–8.

Kulka RA, Schlenger WE, Fairbank JA, Jordan BK, Hough RL, Marmar CR and Weiss DS (1991): Assessment of post-traumatic stress disorder in the community: Prospects and pitfalls from recent studies of Vietnam veterans. *J. Consult. Clin. Psychol* 3: 547–60.

Kumar R and Robson KM (1984): A prospective study of emotional disorders in childbearing women. *British Journal of Psychiatry* 144: 35–47.

Lester D (1995). Preventing suicide in women and men. *Crisis* 16 2: 79–84.

Longobucco DC and Freston MS (1989): Relation of somatic symptoms to degree of paternal-role preparation of first-time expectant fathers. *Journal of Obstetric, Gynaecology and Neonatal Nursing* 18 6: 482–8.

Lovestone S and Kumar RC (1993): Postnatal psychiatric illness: The impact on partners. *British Journal of Psychiatry*. 163: 210–6.

McNall LK (1976): Concerns of Expectant Fathers. In: McNall L and Galeener J (eds): *Current Practice in Obstetrics and Gynaecology*. St Louis: Mosby.

May KA (1982a): Factors contributing to first time fathers' readiness for fatherhood: An explanatory study. *Family Relations* 31: 353–61.

May KA (1982b): The father as observer. *The American Journal of Maternal Child Nursing* 7 3: 319–22.

May KA (1982c): Three phases of father involvement in pregnancy. *Nursing Research* 31: 337–42.

Meldrum L and Raphael B (1995): Hazardous occupations and mental health. In: National Health and Medical Research Council (ed.): *Men and Mental Health*. Canberra: AGPS.

Milgrom J (1994): Mother–infant Interaction. In: Carter J (ed.): *Postnatal Depression: Towards a Research Agenda for Human Services and Health*. Canberra: AGPS, pp. 55–64.

Mitchell JT (1983): When disaster strikes — the critical incident stress debriefing process. *Jems*. January.

Najman JM (1995): Society, Culture and Male Mental Health. In: National Health and Medical Research Council (ed.): *Men and Mental Health*. Canberra: AGPS.

National Health and Medical Research Council (1995): *Men and Mental Health*. Canberra: AGPS.

Ormel J, van den brink W and Koeter MWJ (1990): Recognition, management, and outcome of psychological disorders in primary care: a naturalistic follow-up study. *Psychol. Med.* 20: 909–23.

Orsillo SM, Weathers FW, Litz BT, Steinberg HR, Huska JA and Keane TM (1996): Current and lifetime psychiatric disorders among veterans with war zone-related post-traumatic stress disorder. *Journal of Nervous and Mental Disease* 184 5: 307–13.

Osofsky H (1982): Expectant and new fatherhood as a developmental crisis. *Bulletin of the Menninger Clinic* 46 3: 209–30.

O'Toole AI, Marshall RP, Grayson DA and Schureck RJ (1995): War and Mental Health. In: National Health and Medical Research Council, *Men and Mental Health*. Canberra: AGPS.

Paykel ES and Priest RG (1992): Recognition and management of depression in general practice: Consensus statement. *British Medical Journal* 305: 1198–202.

Phongsavan P, Ward J, Oldenburg BF and Gordon JJ (1995): Mental health care practices and educational needs of general practitioners. *The Medical Journal of Australia* 162: 139–42.

Raphael B (1993): *Scope for Prevention*. Canberra: National Mental Health and Medical Research Council.

Repetti RL (1989): The effects of daily workload on subsequent behaviour during marital interaction: The roles of social withdrawal and spouse support. *Journal of Personality and Social Psychology* 57: 651–9.

Rey J (1992): The Epidemiologic Catchment Area (ECA) Study: Implications for Australia. *Australian and New Zealand Journal of Psychiatry* 24: 323–30.

Rickel A (1984): *Social and Psychological Problems of Women*. New York: Hemisphere Publishers.

Russell G (1983): *The Changing Role of Fathers*. St Lucia, Queensland: University of Queensland Press.

Schoenborn CA and Horm J (1993): Negative moods as correlates of smoking and heavier drinking: Implications for health promotion. *Advance Data from Vital and Health Statistics. No 236.* Hyattsville, Maryland: National Center for Health Statistics.

Seager CP (1960): A controlled study of postpartum mental illness. *Journal of Mental Science* 106: 214–30.

Stein GS (1984): Emotional reactions to childbirth: Maternity blues. *Modern Medicine* 29 2: 31–5.

Swanson J (1980): The marital sexual relationship during pregnancy. *Journal of Obstetric, Gynaecology and Neonatal Nursing* 9 5: 267–70.

Tomlinson B, White MA and Wilson ME (1990): Family dynamics during pregnancy. *Journal of Advanced Nursing* 15: 683–8.

Watson JP, Elliott SA, Rugg AJ and Brough DI (1984): Psychiatric disorder in pregnancy and the postnatal year. *British Journal of Psychiatry* 144: 453–62.

Personal communication

Michael Dudley, November 1997.

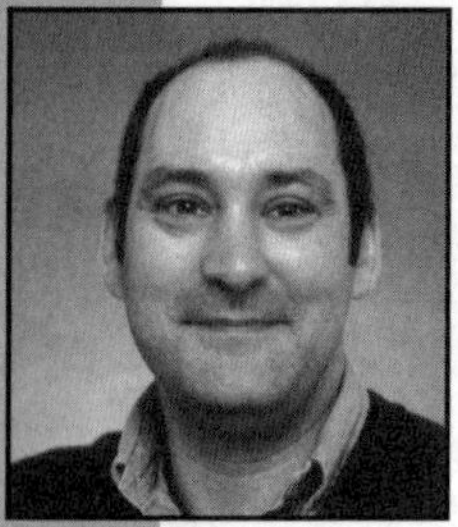

STEPHEN A. HARROP

Registered Nurse, Bachelor of Science, Doctor of Philosophy

Stephen Harrop qualified as a registered nurse in 1980. He underwent hospital-based training at Darwin Hospital in the Northern Territory. He has nursed in a wide variety of areas including remote Australian regions and metropolitan acute care settings. More recently, he completed a Bachelor of Science in bioscience and was awarded his doctorate for studies in tropical health and medical-based molecular biology. His strong interest in the men's movement involves him in a number of Brisbane-based groups.

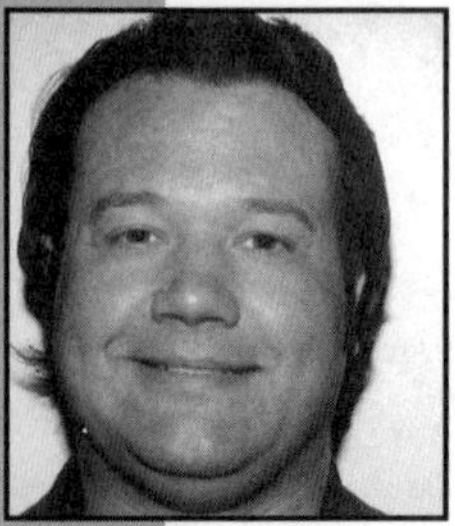

GREGORY J. CAMERON

Bachelor of Nursing

Gregory Cameron qualified recently with a Bachelor of Nursing following a long career of nursing with the Department of Defence. He has extensive practical nursing experience, particularly in areas related to men's health. At present he is a practising nurse at the QEII Hospital and District Health Service in Brisbane and is undertaking an Occupational Health and Safety Graduate Diploma at the Queensland University of Technology.

Chapter 13

Male sterilisation — changing the culture of families

INTRODUCTION

A simple text search of the internet using the word <vasectomy> reveals a plethora of sites, many of which are essentially advertising clinics that undertake vasectomy. The sites may include an information page about

- the procedure,
- when and to whom the procedure would be appropriate, and
- possible health effects.

Superficially, these guides disseminate information. However, this apparently simple answer to the question of male sterilisation seems to be misleading because there appears to be a significant number of men wishing to have their fertility restored using advanced technologies.

Western culture is still predominantly heterosexual revolving around the concept of the nuclear family or extended family. Why then do men present themselves for surgical sterilisation? Does vasectomy relate to the high divorce rate and what is the social impact? Vasectomy is often a taboo topic by virtue of the fact that it is a permanent procedure — a man making a choice about his future fertility. What are the choices then, for a man who enters into a new relationship where children are an expectation?

Because such reproductive decisions impact profoundly upon family life, should preference be given to the values of those who will live with the consequences? (Bartels, 1991). Ethical issues arise when we deal with contraceptive, sterilisation and fertility methods. Are the reproductive technologies driven by commercial factors or are they a service that is client focused? If the technologies are client driven, in what circumstances (born out of social pressures) do the clients present themselves?

REPRODUCTIVE REASONING

The reasons that people wish to retain their fertility are biological, psychological, sociological, economic, cultural and religious. Common statements such as 'we must breed in order to maintain the human race and to pass on the family name' may appear to be rather superficial and altruistic in nature. The real reasons for bringing children into the world, however, may have much deeper underpinnings.

Often romantic notions of parenting arise. Children are seen as the product of a loving sexual union in the family context, that is, fruitful outcome of sexual intercourse. The notion of having a child grows out of a need within the relationship. Potential parents may state that they have 'a long-standing relationship with my unborn and unconceived child'. Potential parents also reason that they wish to 'present the pleasures of my world to my child as I see them'. As has been said, Western culture is strongly heterosexual and remains based around the nuclear and extended families. In this context, children adhere to societal norms as 'chattels' of their parents, allowing the parents to complete their perception of a fulfilled partnership.

Economic reasons also justify childbearing. It may be necessary to maintain a title or family name. In a more biological sense, reproduction is the result of various hormonal and developmental factors. Balancing these organic-type factors within the appropriate sociocultural perspective may be difficult for a family.

Children may fill a number of expectations based upon:

- religious convictions
- cultural expectations
- the need for parenting, which is a strong process in relationships
- social and peer expectations
- the opportunity to nurture life
- parenting needs, which may arise from ego or power issues
- the products of biological and hormonal drives
- economic rationale

Until quite recently, the act of parenting was not only accepted but expected. It is interesting to note that people are now beginning to inquire into the reasons for the procreation of children. In contemporary society, 'altruistic' reasons for parenting may now appear rather facile.

CONTRACEPTIVE OPTIONS FOR MEN

Men do not share the burden of fertility regulation, particularly because of their limited options. However, new male methods of contraception, if reversible, may alter men's willingness to accept or share the responsibility of fertility control (Ringheim, 1993).

Developing forms of male contraception include:

- reversible vas occlusion;
- hormonal means of sperm suppression, based upon androgen injections, implants, and other gonadotrophin-suppressing agents; and
- other drug, vaccine and DNA technologies (Waites, 1993)

At present, however, only two types of options exist for male-specific fertility control:

- those methods that are coitus dependent, such as condom or withdrawal and
- those methods which are permanent, such as vasectomy.

VASECTOMY — THE STATISTICS

It has been estimated that 60 per cent of couples in Australia will choose voluntary sterilisation for contraception in their lifetime (Family Planning Queensland, 1994:1). There are approximately 500 000 vasectomy procedures performed annually in the United States. This is a rate of 10.3 procedures per 1000 men aged 29–to 49 years (Marquette et al., 1991). But that is only half the US rate for tubal ligation procedures for women (Wardell, 1994). In the United Kingdom, however, approximately equal numbers of men and women (13 per cent and 12 per cent respectively within the 16–49-year age group) choose surgical sterilisation (McCormack, 1995). Church and Geller (1989) estimate that a total of 43 million vasectomy procedures have been performed globally.

The failure rate for vasectomy is less than 2 per thousand (as compared to the tubal ligation failure rate of 4 per thousand) and vasectomy has a low rate of surgical complications such as

- haematoma,
- infection,
- epididymytis and
- scrotal pain (Strodl, 1996).

Physicians advise their patients that vasectomy is permanent and irreversible. This has come about because of malpractice suits associated with vasectomy.

At present 8 per cent of urologists in the United States do not perform vasectomy as it has one of the highest malpractice rates for urology procedures. Litigation is due mainly to

- surgical complications arising and
- failure to provide a proper informed consent (Fischman and Nagler, 1991).

Many of the purported health risks associated with vasectomy have been well studied, including the association of vasectomy with prostate cancer and heart disease. Recent large studies have failed to provide a significant link between vasectomy and prostate cancer (John et al.,1995), and vasectomy has not been associated with an increase in overall mortality or mortality from cancer (Giovannuccit et al., 1992). Moreover, psychosocial adjustment of sterilised men is superior to that of nonsterilised men (perhaps due to reduced fear of pregnancy) as assessed through interviews by Janke and Wiest (1976–77). Large, controlled studies of men who have undergone vasectomy have failed to confirm associations and the conclusion can be drawn that

> Vasectomy has no major effects on the physical or mental health of men (Thonneau and D'Isle, 1990).

This viewpoint will now be explored with respect to family issues.

FERTILITY TECHNOLOGIES

Pregnancy follows vasectomy reversal in approximately 50 per cent of cases with higher rates for those who choose reversal within 10 years of vasectomy (Fischman and Nagler, 1991). Although vasectomy reversal is often technically successful (90 per cent), fertility is restored in only 40–70 per cent of cases (Fischman and Nagler, 1991). Failure may occur due to

- the production of sperm antibodies or
- immune cell mediated responses against sperm.

In the US about 10.5 per cent of couples in remarriages seek donor insemination because a reversed vasectomy has not produced fertility (Humphrey and Humphrey, 1993).

The issue of vasectomy producing permanent infertility is being addressed proactively in some countries. For example, a semen storage facility opened by Cryobanks of Florida in the USA in 1996 suggests to men considering vasectomy that they should keep their parenting options open by storing their sperm. In addition, there is a suite of clinics offering assisted reproductive techniques for infertile men, many of which may particularly suit men post-vasectomy. These procedures include

- the sperm-recovery techniques percutaneous epididymal sperm aspiration (PESA) and microepididymal sperm aspiration (MESA),

- gamete intrafallopian transfer (GIFT) and
- a modification of the in vitro fertilisation (IVF) technique, intracytoplasmic sperm injection (ICSI), in which a single sperm is injected into the cytoplasm of an ovum.

In a recent media report (Gorman, 1997), the US National Institutes of Health director, Dr Harold Varmus, told a US congressional subcommittee that just one infertile couple could argue that human cloning provides their only chance to bear a child, and that this may turn public opinion around.

Technologies related to reproduction post sterility:

- sperm cryostorage
- percutaneous epididymal sperm aspiration (PESA)
- microepididymal sperm aspiration (MESA)
- in vitro fertilization (IVF) technique
- gamete intrafallopian transfer (GIFT)
- intracytoplasmic sperm injection (ICSI)
- surrogacy using any of the above technologies
- somatic cell line cloning

A paradox now arises. On one hand, vasectomy is offered on the understanding that the operation will herald the end of their reproductive life, whilst on the other hand, when men present for vasectomy, they may be given advice on sperm banking and post-sterility fertility technology.

Another issue is the use of stored sperm. In a recent media report from the UK, a woman attempted to have access to her deceased husband's semen in order to become pregnant. British legislation covering such matters decreed that this woman could not have the semen because the deceased husband could not give authorisation to release it. In addition, the authorities were unwilling to allow the procedure to go ahead. Eventually, a continental European fertility clinic agreed to perform the procedure. The woman brought the state to court in order to release the sperm to the European clinic. In considering the ethics of this case, there appears a need to protect both parties. Unforeseen circumstances similar in nature to these may present themselves in the future. It is necessary to examine, therefore, who has ownership or access to human gametes, and what or who drives the reproductive technologies.

Fertility technologies are not always sought because of a vasectomy. Approximately 10 per cent of couples who desire pregnancy are infertile, 10–20 per cent of these couples having unexplained infertility (Mandelbaum, 1987). The rate of assisted conception (such as IVF) rises with age of the female partner. For women aged between 20 years and 29 years it is 0.8 per cent, but it increases to 2.2 per cent for 30–34 year olds, and to 3.7 per cent for those older than 35 years (Roberts et al., 1994).

Altruistic and paternal surrogacy issues are increasingly the subject of public debate (Stuhmcke, 1996). Surrogacy may deal with high-level use of reproductive technology. It is also necessary to examine the interpretation of law with respect to adoption, social and ethical paternity and maternity issues. The values of the law with respect to the contemporary family must also be questioned. The wider issue of contraceptive and fertility technologies rests with the owners of the technology and sociological and cultural forces.

WHY MEN PRESENT FOR VASECTOMY

There appear to be at least two types of reasons why men have vasectomy within a family context:

- contraceptive and
- psychosocial.

Vasectomy is a permanent form of contraception. It results from a pragmatic approach to contraception: 'we wish to continue our sex life without fear of pregnancy' or 'because my partner is unable to use contraception due to health, personal or religious reasoning'.

Vasectomy circumvents the need for hormonal, chemical, barrier, and behavioral methods of contraception. It appears, at least superficially, to be a less complicated form of contraception. Indeed, vasectomy presents itself as a safer and less expensive form of fertility control than other forms, both recent and traditional.

Why then is vasectomy, as a contraceptive, sought? More common reasons include 'we have enough children' having reached their utopian ideal family size and 'we do not want children'. Couples who have undergone genetic counselling may choose vasectomy in order to prevent the transmission of potentially devastating and incurable genetic diseases (for example, cystic fibrosis, haemophilia and heritable psychiatric disorders). There is also the issue of trust in contraceptive use — if the male has reason to believe that he cannot rely upon his partner for contraceptive management. There are also issues such as limiting family size (the outcome being population control) and the more subtle 'eugenics by choice'.

Vasectomy is complicated by self-perception. This issue contains family and political consequences. Self-regulation of contraception in the male is viewed as the conscious control of fertility so is a form of self-empowerment. Health professionals may not always consider the underlying psychosocial situation in the client's relationship within his family — the amount of professional insight into a client's psyche is limited by client self-disclosure. Does the male use this power as a lever within the relationship? Is there a strong link between control of contraception and control within the relationship?

Vasectomy is one of the only contraceptive choices that men have access to so its psychosocial and psychosexual underpinnings need to be addressed. The man may say 'I am making this commitment to my family', thus pledging permanence. Sterilisation in this context is used to contribute to the partnership and family. Or it may be an attempt to save a failing relationship. Men who wish to take control of contraceptive matters may be carrying out a protective role with respect to their partner. The newly sterilised male feels happy; he has contributed to the family and it was his decision. However it may alter the direction of the family — permanently.

Other reasons for vasectomy include pressure by the partner not to use a condom or peer group coercion to undergo sterilisation. Men may be swept along by the fervor of peers and colleagues. It is not uncommon for a police station or fire station to go 'vasectomy mad' (McCormack, 1995). The 'vasectomy club motto' is 'Cut now, join tomorrow'.

'Escapers' are those men who undergo vasectomy so that they never have children. These men have a conscientious objection to fathering. They feel idealistically opposed to global overpopulation and are convinced of the unsuitability of the modern world for children (McCormack, 1995). However, while these men challenge the Western belief of parenting they may feel guilty about not living up to societal and cultural norms.

In light of new fertility technology, men may be able to 'keep their options open' but they will become dependent upon the technology process and those who control the access to the technology and the way this technology is used.

OUTCOME — PSYCHOLOGICAL POST-STERILITY PROBLEMS

Elective surgery on the male primary sex organs can greatly affect the male psyche by changing the concepts of self-image, virility, and manliness. For example, a small study of vasectomised men with erectile dysfunction attributed to vasectomy suggested that low acceptance of the vasectomy by a predominant female partner may cause erectile dysfunction (Buchholz et al., 1994).

Post-sterilisation regret encompasses psychosocial concepts of self-image and the image of the partner. It may be necessary for the man to undergo an emotional readjustment about his new role with respect to contraception and the male psyche. The female partner may also undergo an emotional upheaval and this may be expressed as a type of mourning for the loss of fertility in her partner. This is not unlike the mourning the loss of fertility at menopause.

According to Miller et al. (1991), those most likely to suffer post vasectomy regret are:

- relatively young couples,
- those having ambivalence about future childbearing,
- those with negative attitudes towards sterilisation and
- those who experience conflict during decision making.

Remarriage in Australia is now more common and is linked to the increasing divorce rate (see below). Approximately 10.5 per cent of vasectomised men request reversal due to a new family situation (Humphrey and Humphrey, 1993). These data indicate a need for improving pre-sterilisation education and counselling.

THE IMPACT OF STERILISATION ON THE FAMILY

In Australia, the 1995 marriage rate for those of 15 years or older was 36.7 per 1000 for men and 36.0 per 1000 for women. Interestingly, the divorce rate for the same year was 12.3 per 1000 marriages, compared with a rate of 10.9 per 1000 marriages in 1985. The median duration of marriage in Australia in 1995 was 7.6 years, with 42.9 per cent of all marriages ending in divorce (McLennan, 1995).

Clearly these data indicate some disharmony within Australian relationships. When compared to the rates of vasectomy and those seeking vasectomy reversal, it may be suggested that vasectomy is an unquantifiable but real component of family statistics. In what way can partners understand each other's point of view on the matter of sterilisation? How can they reach an agreement on sterilisation?

Family health information may be obtained from general medical practitioners and community health centres. More specific information can be found at family planning clinics. However, men in particular obtain health information from less formal sources. These include

- 'mates' who have dealt with some of these issues or experiences,
- partners,
- print media (especially women's and family magazines) and, occasionally,
- television reports.

In Britain, in a study of a gynaecologist's case notes of women undergoing sterilisation, only 22 per cent mentioned the option of vasectomy (Penney et al., 1997). In Ireland, where comprehensive counselling given at a family planning clinic was a mandatory prerequisite of vasectomy, the majority of men (99 per cent) were pleased with the procedure and did not suffer complications

(Orr and Moore, 1989). It has been suggested that any organisation which includes vasectomy in its program of family planning should include advice and referral for vasectomy reversal (Hendry, 1994). On standard vasectomy consent forms, reversal technology is not suggested, neither is the option of sperm banking (see Figure 13.1).

Figure 13.1 Standard contemporary vasectomy consent form

(Note that vasectomy is presented as a permanent form of contraception and that reversal technology is not mentioned. Similarly, sperm banking prior to the procedure is not suggested.)

VASECTOMY CONSENT FORM

I, ______________________________, authorise

Dr______________________________ to perform a VASECTOMY, which consists of the surgical removal of a segment of the vas deferens (the tube that conveys sperm from the testicles to the outside).

Other methods of treatment, including not having this procedure done, have been discussed with me and I have chosen this method. I understand the following:

1. That the purpose of a vasectomy is to render me permanently sterile.
2. That there is no guarantee that sterility will be obtained (sterility is either not obtained or
fertility returns in approximately one case in five hundred).
3. That possible complications include, but are not limited to:

- pain
- swelling
- possible psychological effect on my sex life
- bleeding
- infection
- allergy to local anesthetic
- failure to achieve permanent sterilisation
- vas deferens may grow back together in the first few months or later.

4. That I must continue to use contraceptives until sterility is confirmed by the doctor after two sperm counts.

I have had an opportunity to ask questions and have had them answered. In addition, I have read this form and it has been explained to me in lay terminology. I understand the risks and intend to have the procedure done.

Date ____________________

Signature ______________________________

Witness ______________________________

Spouse, if applicable, ______________________________

DOCTOR'S STATEMENT: The patient and I have discussed this procedure, including its risks and complications, and we have discussed alternatives. To the best of my knowledge, the patient understands the procedure and consents to it.

(Doctor's signature) ______________________________

Date ____________________

The process of dealing with the issue of sterilisation in the family runs the gamut of the communication spectrum. From a rational, informed and open discussion, communication can be reduced to a curt settlement or a one-way uncompromising trade-off that leads to unilateral decision-making. For example, men do not always get consent from their partners and usually not from future partners. It is obvious then, that when vasectomy is being considered, the question of who should consent must also be considered.

A number of issues may arise out of sterilisation:

Trust

An issue of trust relates to an issue of promiscuity. The woman may feel that vasectomy can imply potential promiscuity. It may conjure up a notion of infidelity, real or imagined, between partners now that fertility per se is no longer an issue. There is also the male issue of not trusting the woman with contraception. When there is no contraception issue within the partnership, the vasectomy may be used as a contraceptive outside of the partnership.

Future relationships

There is also the concern for any future relationships in which children may be desired. When a female partner is involved in the consent process, the male may feel resentment if he enters a new relationship. It is difficult for a health professional to make clear to a vasectomy candidate that the procedure may not be good for possible future relationships but the issue must be canvassed.

Sexual health

Though fertility is usually the primary issue in vasectomy, infection issues that were previously dealt with by condoms are still relevant. The vasectomised male who has an affair may be less inclined to use a condom and so can bring disease into the partnership. Sexually transmitted diseases need to be dealt with using conventional methods.

In general, women are believed to approach the issues of childlessness and infertility on an emotional level, whilst men may approach the issue more pragmatically. However, these perceived attitudes may reflect social and cultural expectations. Childless people should be able to feel fulfilled just as those who have children feel fulfilled. This is a view put forward by discussants of reproductive technologies. They express the notion that women may have a fulfilling life without children, but this is not without social pressures (Ewing, 1992).

The notion of male sterilisation is a gender issue on many fronts. Women may go on the oral contraceptive pill in their early teens, but males of the same age have no option, essentially, but to choose condoms. Family planning clinics are now more accessible to men than in previous generations and men are now being proactive in the area of fertility regulation and sexual education. New technologies may thus change the gender focus on fertility.

Men's awareness of contraceptive issues will allow conscious positive decision-making (for example, see the male issues internet link in the reference list at the end of the chapter). Men ask:

- Who can have a vasectomy?
- Is it in the control of the surgeon?
- To what extent can one take control of one's biology and thus take responsibility for contraception?

These questions are asked in the light of the statistics of non-paternity within marriages. In Australia, of those couples who present for paternity testing (for whatever reason), between 10 and 25 per cent of cases return a nonpaternity finding (*XY Men*, 1996:7). This data may be skewed towards cases involving paternity issues, such as child residency conflicts, or in cases of claims for paternal maintenance and government family benefit. The incidence of nonpaternity is generally thought to be between 10 and 15 per cent, with 10 per cent a widely quoted figure in textbooks (MacIntyre and Sooman, 1991).

ETHICAL CONSIDERATIONS

There is a need to increase the profile of health education for men, particularly sex education, because men as a group have not previously shared equally with women in fertility regulation. The general issues of global fertility are sometimes addressed by governments. The Indian government suggested that a portable radio be given to every man undergoing a vasectomy. Some other nations, for example Bangladesh, offer small monetary incentives. The Chinese government appears more coercive and promotes the 'one family one child program' by applying higher tax levies for larger families and treating larger families as social outcasts by restricting their access to community services. Family size and fertility in the Western world, however, are in part driven by economic factors — children are expensive.

Global fertility and population issues relate, to some extent, to the availability, cost and marketing of products from multinational pharmaceutical and medical companies as well as to the accessibility of medical technologies. The World Health Organization also directs various contraceptive campaigns. One must now ask:

- 'Who is responsible for population control?', and
- 'What ethical issues need addressing when there is an alteration of the fertility of peoples?

It is especially important to respect the culture and social wellbeing of all peoples when dealing with global fertility issues.

DUTY OF THE HEALTH CARE PROFESSIONAL

The aim of the physician is to minimise the psychosexual and immediate post-operative complications and the number of reversal requests after vasectomy (Linnet, 1983). The role of the nursing professional must encompass the holistic approach. The nurse aims to ensure that the person undergoing sterilisation is given

- relevant information, that is, all information about sterilisation and pre- and post-sterilisation options (such as the storage of sperm),
- encouragement of self expression, and, particularly,
- advocacy.

Value statement 3.3 of the Australian Nursing Council Incorporated (1993) encourages nursing professionals to act as an advocate when the rights of the individual are overlooked. In light of new and developing technologies and the relationship of science and medicine in Western countries, the question of rights today and in the future, becomes paramount (Johnstone, 1994). As explored earlier in this chapter, law and ethics need to be examined as a continuum. That is, the health professional must stay informed about established, new and future forms of reproductive technologies, so that those considering vasectomy (and their families) can be sure of the appropriate guidance.

Acknowledgments

The authors wish to thank the Family Planning Clinic of Queensland in Fortitude Valley, and Jenny A. Fraser for her useful comments and discussions.

References

Australian Nursing Council Incorporated (1993): *National Competencies for the Registered Nurses and Enrolled Nurses in Recommended Domains.* Canberra, ACT, p 9.

Bartels D (1991): genetic counseling: Ethics, values and professional responsibilities. *Human Genome News* 3: 1–2. (http://www.ornl.gov/TechResources/Human_Genome/publicat/hgn/v3n2/14bartel.html)

Buchholz NP, Weuste R, Mattarelli G, Woessmer B and Langewitz W (1994): Post-vasectomy erectile dysfunction. *Journal of Psychosomatic Research* 38: 759–762.

Church CA and Geller J (1989): Lights! Camera! Action! Promoting family planning with TV, video, and film. *Population and Reproduction Journal* 38: 2–31.

Ewing C (1992): *Manufacturing Babies.* Canberra: National Women's Consultative Council.

Family Planning Queensland (1994): Voluntary sterilisation information sheet. December: 1.

Fischman M and Nagler HM (1991): New options for vasectomy. *Medical Aspects of Human Sexuality*: 33–38.

Giovannuccit E, Tosteson TD, Speizer FE, Vessey MP, and Colditz GA (1992): A long-term study of men who have undergone vasectomy. *New England Journal of Medicine* 326: 1392–1398.

Gorman G [reporter] (1997): Neti and Ditto, two cute new clones are too close for comfort. *Time Magazine*: 11, 111.

Hendry WF (1994): Vasectomy and vasectomy reversal. *British Journal of Urology* 73: 337–344.

Humphrey M and Humphrey H (1993): Vasectomy as a reason for donor insemination. *Social Science and Medicine* 37: 263–266.

Janke L and Wiest WM (1976–77) Psychosocial and medical effects of vasectomy in a sample of health plan subscribers. *International Journal of Psychiatric Medicine* 7: 17–34.

John EM, Whittmore AS, Wu AH, Kolonel LN, Hislop TG, Howe GR, West DW, Hankin J, Dreon DM and Teh CZ (1995): Vasectomy and prostate cancer: Results from a multiethnic case-control study. *Journal of the National Cancer Institute* 87: 662–669.

Johnstone M-J (1994): *Bioethics a Nursing Perspective*, 2nd edn. Sydney: WB Saunders Bailliere Tindall, p. 270.

Linnet L (1983) Clinical immunology of vasectomy and vasovasostomy. *Urology* XXII: 101–112.

McCormack D (1995): Vasectomy — is it on enough agendas? *British Journal of Sexual Medicine* 22: 13–15.

MacIntyre S and Sooman A (1991): Non-paternity and prenatal genetic screening. *Lancet* 338: 869–871.

McLennan (1995). *Marriages and Divorces, Australia*. Catalogue no. 3310.0 Canberra: Australian Bureau of Statistics, pp. 5–75.

Male issues internet link: http://www.ozemail.com.au/~irgeo

Mandelbaum SL, Diamond MP and Deterrent AH (1987): The impact of antiserum antibodies on human infertility. *Journal of Urology* 138:1–8.

Marquette CM, Koonin LM, Antarsh L, Gargiullo PM and Smith JC (1991): Vasectomy in the United States. *American Journal of Public Health* 85: 644–649.

Miller B, Shain RN and Pasta DJ (1991): The predictors of post-sterilization regret in married women. *Journal of Applied Sociology and Psychology* 21: 1083–1110.

Orr D and Moore B (1989): Vasectomy as a contraceptive method. *Irish Medical Journal* 82: 19–20.

Penney GC, Souter V, Glasier A and Templton AA (1997): Laparascopic sterilisation: opinion and practice among gynaecologists in Scotland. *The British Journal of Obstetrics and Gynaecology* 104: 71–77.

Ringheim K (1993): Factors that determine prevalence of use of contraceptive methods for men. *Studies in Family Planning* 24: 87–99.

Roberts, Christine L, Algert, Charles S and March, Lyn M (1994): Delayed childbearing — are there any risks? *The Medical Journal of Australia* 160: 539–544.

Strodl E (1996): Voluntary Surgical Sterilisation In: *A Review of Men's Health Literature*. Darling Downs Regional Health Authority: Health Promotion Unit, pp. 93–96.

Stuhmcke A (1996): For love or money: The legal regulation of surrogate motherhood. E Law — Murdoch University Electronic Journal of Law 3 1. (http://www.murdoch.edu.au/elaw/issues/v3n1/stuhmck1.html)

Thonneau P and D'Isle B (1990): Does vasectomy have long-term effects on somatic and psychological health status? *International Journal of Andrology* 13: 419–432.

Waites GM (1993): Male fertility regulation: The changes for the year 2000. *British Medical Bulletin* 49: 210–221.

Wardell DW (1994): Commentary on long-term consequences of female and male sterilization. *AWHONNS Women's Health Nursing Scan* 8: 10–11.

XY Men (1996), Spring, p. 7, report taken from the *Canberra Times*, 18 February 1996.

Suggested reading

McLennan (1994). *Marriages and Divorces, Australia*. Catalogue no. 3310.0 Part A: Special Feature, How many marriages end in divorce? Canberra: Australian Bureau of Statistics, pp. 9–14.

Section Four

CURRENT ISSUES — THE LIVED EXPERIENCE

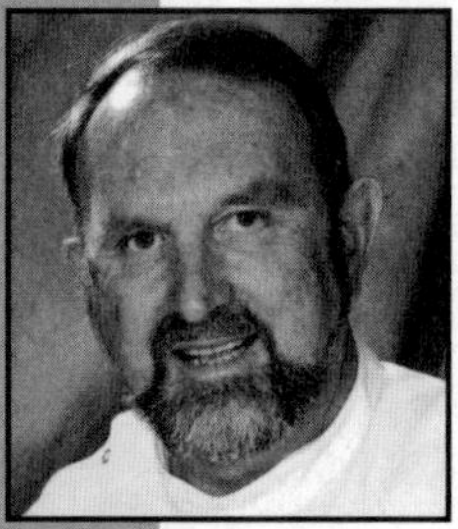

GRAHAM CRAPP

Graham Crapp is a graduate of Sydney University, a Fellow of the Australian Institute of Pharmacy Marketing and a member of the Royal Pharmaceutical Society of Great Britain. Until 30 June 1998, he was a practising consultant pharmacist and a partner in Wodonga Pharmacy. He lectures part-time in marketing at Wodonga Institute of TAFE. In March 1997 Graham was elected Mayor of the City of Wodonga, Victoria's fastest-growing city. Graham is married to an artist and potter and has three sons in their early 20s. He is a level 2 ski instructor (and passionate about skiing), a keen sailor and loves spending time with people. Graham has had a long involvement in adult education and is always keen to share his experiences, especially in the areas of communication, leadership and marketing.

Chapter 14

'You have prostate cancer.'

It's a crisp, sunny winter day in the northeast of Victoria, a day that induces a rare feeling of wellbeing. Standing in the sunshine beside a window in a crowded waiting room I hear my name called. I walk briskly towards the consulting room, confident of good news. Looking past the specialist to the first wattle blossoms of the winter. I hear the words, 'I'm sorry, your biopsy was positive. You have prostate cancer.'

Nine years earlier I had presented to my GP with urinary tract problems. Occasionally I experienced pain on ejaculation and a soreness at the end of the penis whilst urinating. This feeling would last for a week or two and then disappear and at no stage was it affecting my lifestyle. It was just mildly irritating. My GP correctly diagnosed prostatitis, a term used to describe various forms of inflammation of the prostate. Chronic bacterial prostatitis (CBP) had become a way of life over the next few years. CBP is not life-threatening — the symptoms can be treated but they cannot be eliminated. The complex number of little tubes and sacs in the prostate make it very difficult for medication to penetrate into every part of the gland. Infection almost always lies dormant, waiting for the right time to flare up. In 1994 a Prostate Sensitive Antigen (PSA) test showed a very slight elevation from the norm and I agreed with my GP that it was probably caused by the CBP. PSA is a glycoprotein, detectable in the blood, which is found exclusively in the prostate and is present in a very high percentage of prostate cancers.

In February 1995 I joined two of my sons in Canada to participate in an intensive eight-week, level 2 ski instructors course. Despite being 55 years of age, I managed to keep up with the (mainly) 20-year olds and to pass the final examinations. I found that skiing at Blackcomb in the beautiful Garibaldi

current information. Incidentally, I still use this source to keep abreast of the latest developments. And then I had my first stroke of good luck. My mother had discovered in her local library a copy of a book called *Prostate Cancer: Making Survival Decisions* by Sylvan Meyer and Seymour Nash. It provides a wealth of current information on every aspect of prostate cancer. At the time, July 1995, the copy in my mother's library was the only copy in Australia and it took nearly three months to obtain my own copy from America. It is now available in limited quantities from Dymocks. This book is a must for all men diagnosed with prostate cancer and, dare I say, should be compulsory reading for every urologist. As I waded through the reading I found very few areas of consensus and I began to compile a list of questions that needed answering. I felt that I needed at least one more opinion.

For several months I had been following the fortunes of a close friend who had opted for a relatively new form of treatment for prostate cancer called cryotherapy. Put simply cryotherapy involves freezing the affected prostate and destroying the cancerous tissue. This is done by inserting small tubes through the patient's crotch and into the prostate and filling them with liquid nitrogen. The treatment had been successful for my friend and he was impressed by the noninvasive form of the surgery. So the only urologist currently using this system was high on my list of people to talk to. I also found a urology specialist in Melbourne to whom I could relate and in whom I had great confidence.

As I talked to each of these men I summoned all my powers of concentration and if there was something that I didn't understand I kept asking questions. I had to be very confident that I was making the best decision and that I had complete faith and trust in the person who would finally undertake any surgery. I am absolutely certain that a large part of the successful treatment of cancer involves a profound belief in the decisions that you make, which includes faith and confidence in your specialist.

This is the list of questions that I asked each urologist:

1. Can you please explain where my prostate is and what its function is? Can you please explain what type of cancer prostate cancer is? Does it grow quickly?
2. Do I need to act swiftly in deciding what course of action to take? How long can I wait before deciding on a course of treatment?
3. At my age what are the threats to my quality of life and what are my chances of dying of prostate cancer before something else gets me?
4. What is the stage of my cancer? (Broadly speaking, 'staging' classifies the location and spread, if any, of the cancer.)
5. What is the Gleeson grade of my cancer?
6. What is the 'ploidy' of my tumour?

(I needed to know the answer to these last three questions in order to discuss my cancer with each specialist. I took great care and a lot of study to know just what each one meant but it is not important to understand fully each system of grading.)

7. What has been the experience of other men with readings similar to mine for PSA, the Gleeson grade and the 'ploidy' of the tumour?
8. What are the treatment methods for prostate cancer?
9. What is the best treatment, or combination of treatments, for me? Is watchful waiting an option?
10. What is the probability of cure, mortality, complications and other side effects of the treatment which seems best suited to me?
11. What are the downsides of treatment relative to my quality of life, including treatment of possible side effects and the possibility of complete impotence?
12. What is the possibility of incontinence in the short and the long term?
13. Is it possible to cure prostate cancer?
14. What are the chances that the diagnosis and the staging of the cancer may be different? What happens if they are?
15. Where can I obtain more information?
16. Are there any counselling services?
17. What happens if, after treatment, my cancer reappears? Which initial procedure is most likely to avoid recurrence? Which offers the best chance for a second attempt if the cancer reappears?

Before I could make a final decision about the best method of treatment I had to complete two more tests aimed at deciding how widespread the cancer had become. If prostate cancer has spread (metastasised) outside the prostate capsule it is quite likely to appear in the bone structure. I had a bone scan which showed no spread of the cancer. I then had a computer axial tomography x-ray or 'cat' scan (it x-rays 'slices' of the body) of all my other organs and again no cancer was found. This meant that almost certainly the cancer was confined to the prostate capsule itself.

It is hard to explain the tension that you feel as you go through these tests. A good percentage of diagnosed prostate cancer has metastasised before it is detected and if the cancer has moved beyond the prostate capsule there is no possibility of a 'cure'.

I flew to Sydney to discuss cryotherapy. I found Australia's only (at that stage) cryotherapy urologist to be a delightful caring man who spent nearly an hour explaining the procedures, the likely results and the possible challenges. Here was a person that I could relate to and, although we touched on the subject of a radical prostatectomy (complete removal of the prostate) only for a few minutes, I knew that I would be perfectly happy to let this urologist operate on me.

A few days later my GP made arrangements to accompany me to Melbourne to obtain the opinion of the urologist in whom I had great confidence. I'm sure that having my own GP attend the interview had no bearing on the fact that this person was another genuine, caring physician with whom I could communicate easily and who gave me a feeling of great confidence. We discussed all the possibilities, including cryotherapy, and finally the specialist said, 'If I perform a radical prostatectomy I will have the prostate in my hand and I will know, after a pathology test, just where you stand. I believe radical prostatectomy is your only option.'

During the long drive home I discussed with my GP all the possibilities and all the research that we had done over the last few weeks. Cryotherapy is very much less intrusive than a radical prostatectomy, requires only a few days in hospital and does not interfere with continence. Unfortunately there is no way of knowing that all of the cancer has been destroyed by the freezing process. Because the urethra has to be protected by a tube containing warm water, the tissue close to the urethra cannot be destroyed. Post-operatively it is necessary to continue to have regular PSA and TRUS tests — not a pleasant thought. I discarded cryotherapy on the basis that I would find it difficult to live with the fact that I might have some active prostate cancer no matter how small. Some men don't find that a problem and for many of them the emerging option of cryotherapy offers a very good alternative. A radical prostatectomy seemed to be the only way to go since I had discarded radiation therapy from the very beginning. Tests had shown that there was little likelihood of the cancer having spread and there was every possibility that all the cancerous tissue would be removed. At the rest stop on the Hume Highway near Euroa I announced to my GP that I was going to have a 'radical'.

Elisabeth, my wife and companion for nearly 30 years, had arranged for our three sons to spend the weekend before my operation at home. We are a very close family and we were able to have some sensible discussions about the future . . . including, I might add, who would inherit the family vehicles if I didn't make it! Lis and I then spent the next three days travelling in the countryside and enjoying some very special moments. On 13 November, the night before I was due to report to St Vincents Hospital in Melbourne, Elisabeth and I dined out, saw the film *The Bridges of Madison County* and very tenderly made love for what we knew may well be the last time. Those few days will always be special for us.

The 8th floor of St Vincents Hospital is run by angels. From the time I arrived until they said goodbye, I was cared for meticulously, fussed over and loved! It was my first experience of modern nursing and I was impressed with the professionalism and the skill of the nursing staff.

Waking after a long intense operation is a miracle. Oblivious to a thousand tubes, a catheter, oxygen bottles etc., my only thought was 'I'm alive'. Elisabeth told me that the specialist was pleased with the operation. He confirmed a few days later that the cancer had been confined to the prostate capsule and that it had been short of the margin. (If the cancer is close to the margin of the surgeon's cut there is a possibility that some cancer cells may be on the other side.) I could look forward to a long and happy life.

Modern nursing is so good that within two days I was showering with my catheter and walking around the corridors, not entirely free from pain but almost . . . again because of the wonderful nursing skills of the angels on the 8th floor.

Ten days later I accompanied my catheter home. On 1 December I made this note in my diary:

At exactly 12.07 p.m. on 30 November 1995 I had my catheter removed. I have climbed high mountains and looked out over the world, skied down glaciers in wild and remote regions, canoed exciting rivers, made love in wild and exotic places, watched my sons born, and travelled the world, but nothing beats the sheer joy and exhilaration of having one's catheter removed. At exactly 7.31 this morning, 1 December, less than 24 hours after the removal of the catheter, I had a long, sustained and fairly well-controlled pee. God bless Dr John Moran, my GP; God bless my surgeon; God bless the group of angels (nurses) at St Vincents Private Hospital; and thank God for the wonders of the human body.

Recuperation is a long and slow process. I have learnt to be patient and to overcome the frustration of not being as vigorous as I was before the operation. I think it will probably take me at least another year before I am as fit as I was when I returned from Canada.

It took me exactly a year after the operation to become fully continent and now, more than two years later, I am well on the wayu to becoming fully potent again. On both these counts I have a great deal to thank my highly skilled surgeon for. How do you repay someone who has had such a profound effect on your life?

Facing mortality has greatly enriched my life and I have found a new way of using the experience of having a radical prostatectomy. I joined a prostate support group almost as soon as I was home. I found the frank and open discussion with other men, and the genuine concern they showed for my welfare, very reassuring, and I realised that I had a wonderful opportunity on a daily basis to share my experiences with other men, and to help where possible. Almost every day in the counselling room at the pharmacy I talk to men and their wives about the alternative ways of treating prostate cancer. I talk to them about incontinence and how to cope with the many and various aids that are on the marker (I've tried them all!). I share my experience in hospital and, during the immediate recovery period, I talk to the men about their potency. Most often I channel them into the proper professional area. What I do know is that just being able to talk things through, to explore the possibilities and to know that they are talking to someone who has recovered and has experienced all the trauma is very reassuring. I find this extension of my professional life very fulfilling indeed.

If you ever hear the words 'You have prostate cancer' take heart. It is slow moving. You have plenty of time to make a decision. Don't let anyone rush you. Seek at least two opinions. Find someone to look after you who has a genuine concern, is a good communicator and in whom you have absolute faith. It is quite likely that, as happened for me, the process of facing mortality, reviewing your life and recovering, will leave you a much more fulfilled person with a richer and happier life ahead, no matter how long that might be.

Michael realised that there was nothing else for it but to see the GP. Unfortunately his family GP was on holidays. The replacement doctor saw him briefly and gave him antibiotics, believing it was probably an infection. The prospect of testicular cancer, although remote, could not be excluded and it was arranged for Michael to have an ultrasound.

Michael was impressed by the relaxed demeanour of the female technician who scanned his testicles with a probe. Although he felt a bit awkward at the time he reflected upon the fact that women regularly have tests to assess the health status of their reproductive system. He could see the screen throughout the procedure and the technician pointed out some differences and then went to refer her findings to the radiologists. That evening he came to the kitchen table with a bill and popped it in front of his mother. The item was 'cost of ultra sound: testicular'. His mother responded, 'Is there something that we should know about?' Michael explained to me that, although his family get along very well, it is not usual to broach such personal issues. He explained to his mother that there was a small problem but it was probably nothing to worry about.

The next day he revisited the GP and handed him a sealed envelope from the radiologist. Although Michael was keen to know what had been causing the symptoms he was not prepared for the news he was about to hear. The doctor opened the letter and told him he had cancer and that it had to be removed as soon as possible. The GP's immediate advice was that he should try and stay positive. Michael's reply was 'Give me something to be positive about and I will be.' The GP called around for people he knew who could manage the case. Fortunately Michael could see one surgeon immediately provided he made it across town to the surgeon's rooms within half an hour. By this time Michael was in no fit state to make that destination in the next 25 minutes so he called into Elise's house. He doesn't recall how he got there or how he broke the news, he only remembers being a mess and feeling an overwhelming sense of relief at seeing someone who cared for him and could support him. He made a quick call to his parents, again playing down the news.

Just before 6 o'clock he and Elise entered the waiting room. Michael then saw the surgeon alone. His overwhelming impression of this meeting was that the surgeon was brilliant. He explained the procedure, the type of cancer and the cure rate among the types of cancer. He phoned Michael's parents and then said, 'There is a young lady out there, should she know about this?' Michael answered yes and the surgeon then explained it all to Elise.

The preparation prior to surgery was extensive, involving blood tests, then a body scan to assess if the cancer had spread to other organs. After the operation, which involved the removal of the affected testicle, a pathologist viewed this tissue under a microscope to see if the cancer had infiltrated surrounding tissue.

I asked Michael what his feelings were in relation to having a testicle missing when he woke from the anaesthetic. He replied, 'Well, I wasn't too worried at first, just as long as the cancer was gone. My (step)dad wanted to really reassure me that I would not be "less of a man", and, while I really must say it doesn't worry me, I am glad that I still have one left.' One of Michael's favourite stories to friends and family on his return home from hospital was 'my dog, while being very sympathetic, would gently remind me that things could have been worse — he's lost both!'

After the operation the surgeon informed Michael that the cancer had indeed moved into the lymph glands and that, following a discussion with colleagues , he was recommending chemotherapy. As the surgeon began speaking about the regime of treatment and the side effects of therapy Michael suddenly realised the implications. He was going to be sterile. 'That hit really hard; the whole idea of not having children I was not prepared for.' Michael told me that the idea that, although there was an 80–90 per cent cure rate, he could die, was a lot easier to come to terms with than the fact that he would not be able to have children.

Michael was offered the option of storing his sperm in a sperm bank but was told that there might not be much point as his sperm count was likely to be very low due to the cancer. However, just before his first course of chemotherapy, Michael went to donate his sperm — he felt there was nothing to lose! He said, 'They don't really tell you very much before you get there. Apparently there are these rules, one of them is that you shouldn't ejaculate for 7 days before a deposit.' There should also be gaps between the first and second donation to ensure a good sperm count. However, Michael was very pushed to meet this time frame before he began the chemotherapy schedule.

He remembered his visit to the sperm bank quite clearly; the winding little corridors somewhere at the back of the hospital and a young woman at the desk. He didn't know quite what to say: 'Hi! I'm Michael and . . . I've. . . err . . . got an appointment'. He noted how relaxed and cool the staff were about the whole thing. He was given a specimen jar and escorted to a very nicely furnished room, given his instruction and wished 'good luck'. In fact his luck was in as he later found that although the count was low the sperm were motile.

For chemotherapy he would go into hospital on Thursday morning and come out on Saturday. The 48 hours of chemotherapy happened three times. The first time Michael had the therapy, ate a meal and felt fine. He thought 'This is going to be a breeze.' An hour after the meal he vomited and didn't stop for three days. He couldn't even keep down the medication to prevent vomiting. The anti-emetic injections also had no effect. Although he really wanted to be with Elise and said her support and strength had been amazing, he couldn't handle any noise or movement — the effects of the therapy made him extremely agitated. Even talking to her was an effort. He didn't realise until well after the chemotherapy just how difficult this phase had been for those around him.

Although he had lost his hair he didn't really feel out of place as many young people have cropped hair these days. Michael had lost his hair at the same time a 'Crop a cop' charity drive was taking place. People would donate money if a policeman shaved his head. Whilst shopping one day he was asked by two shop assistants if he was a policeman. Michael felt that losing his hairline was in fact a lot less distressing than losing the hair on his chest. 'After all,' he said, 'you have to wait years for that masculine feature.' Not having to shave, he decided, was a real plus.

At the time we were talking, it was four months since Michael had finished the chemotherapy and returned to work. He doesn't talk to people there about his experiences because he feels that they have little knowledge of cancer and its effects. He does, however, find talking to the people at his local church very beneficial, as the congregation is comprised mainly of old people who have themselves experienced, or cared for, someone with cancer. They understand and can empathise with Michael about his experience. What Michael found interesting was the falling away of contact with his younger friends with whom, prior to the operation, he had spent most of his time. It was the older people from the church, those with whom he had had little to do previously, who sent flowers and cards and stayed in contact.

To keep a check on his general health Michael will have regular blood tests, chest and abdominal x-rays and a CAT scan. He claims that he is getting quite good at drinking the 500–750 ml of contrast medium for the abdominal x-ray.

Michael is still debating with himself how best to educate young men and boys about this potential health problem and is taking a keen interest in men's health issues from here on.

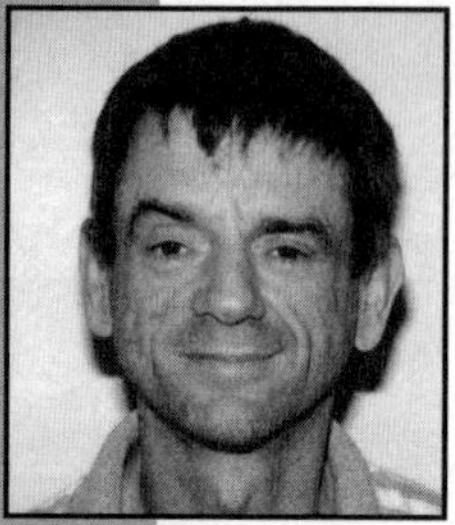

DAVID MENADUE

Bachelor of Arts, Diploma of Education

David Menadue was a teacher and publications officer with the Victorian Department of Education until taking ill-health retirement in 1991. He has been very involved with volunteer work for the Victorian AIDS Council, including holding the posts of Vice-President of the Council and Convenor of People Living with HIV/AIDS Victoria for a number of years. He was instrumental in setting up the Positive Living Centre in St Kilda, a community centre for people with HIV/AIDS. He was awarded an Order of Australia Medal in 1995 for services to the HIV community.

Chapter 16

SURVIVING HIV/AIDS

The first time I was hospitalised for an AIDS-defining illness in 1989 was one of the scariest episodes of my life. It wasn't because of the medical or nursing care at Melbourne's Fairfield Hospital, which was probably amongst the best in the country at the time. It wasn't because of the physical pain and discomfort I was experiencing, although the condition I was admitted for — Pneumocystis Carinii Pneumonia (PCP), a common and often deadly AIDS illness, with high fevers, night sweats and shortness of breath — was certainly making life unpleasant. No, it was a scary experience because of the mental traumas I went through during my time in the hospital ward.

Although I had been aware I was HIV-positive since 1984 and had certainly felt that I had been dealing with the experience reasonably well in the intervening years, the shock of being told that I actually now had 'full-blown' AIDS, was to induce a mental reaction which shocked and surprised me: I guess I didn't realise quite what the human mind is capable of when it is under extreme duress.

My temporary psychotic experience — which is the way, I later discovered, it is described in my medical files — began, not surprisingly, on discovering that the tests for PCP had come back positive and I indeed did now have AIDS. I shouldn't really have been so surprised: plenty of my friends were coming down with the illness's many-varied conditions and I had known for a long time that my T-cells were in the 'danger zone' (below 200). I guess, though, that I had kidded myself, right up until the last minute, that I would not actually develop AIDS and would remain one the charmed few whose health seemed unaffected by the virus.

So many thoughts rushed through my mind as I tried to accommodate my new diagnosis. I first had to ring my parents in northern Victoria and do what I had been too cowardly to do for the past five years: to tell them that I was gay and HIV-positive and now had AIDS. The stress of ringing up my mother and hitting her with this 'double whammy' about my sexuality and my health at a time when I was seriously ill physically was probably what set off the madness which was to follow.

Lying in hospital bed that night I remember hearing lots of banging and thumping happening in the room opposite. It later turned out to be just a noisy pan room but at the time I decided I was opposite a morgue where all the bodies were being dragged during the night. My fevered head pictured the corridors outside awash with blood with the nurses frantically trying to cope with all the death and mayhem about them.

The worst aspect about it all, though, was that somehow I was the cause of this sudden upswing in mortality which had afflicted the hospital. Since I had been admitted to the hospital, I decided, people were starting to 'fall like flies'. I would hear a groan or a sigh in a nearby room: oh yes, another one's gone! And, even more horrifying, I could put the curse of death on people just by looking at them: one glance from my little eye and people who walked into my room, be it nurses or just friends visiting, could be in mortal danger. (Never mind that when I did actually build up the courage to look people in the eye in this state of mind, it didn't happen! Such inconsistencies didn't seemed to register in my disturbed mind.)

Obviously the hospital would have to get rid of this horrible agent of death who had appeared in their midst, this patient whose very presence was somehow causing others to depart the mortal coil. In the middle of the night three or four nurses would be standing around my bed (obviously wondering they could do to quell my bizarre behaviour) and I would be wondering which one of them was hiding the hypodermic which was going to be used to get rid of me and allow the hospital to go back to more normal, peaceful times.

One night I was going to die. I'd felt a levitation feeling which indicated that I was on my way upwards to Heaven's Pearly Gates. While I was ready for this turn of events, I wanted to see my family before I went and, horror of horrors, the hospital wasn't letting them in to see me. They had set up barricades outside the ward, with police and firemen and the like all stopping my relatives from getting in to pay their last respects! Somehow a closed-circuit television had been set up for me and, in what was to be my last moments on earth, I was able to see each of my brothers and sisters and my mother and father one last time before I died.

I am not suggesting that all people who develop AIDS have similar mental experiences to this on diagnosis though I do know that other friends have also had a disturbing time whilst taking heavy doses of the drug Bactrim used to treat PCP. I have since been found to have an allergy to the drug and it is quite possible that this contributed to the severity of these mental symptoms.

I am relating all this mental turmoil here, embarrassing as it is to reveal to others, because I think it shows some of the deep feelings of stigma and guilt which I had developed in my subconscious over the years of living with HIV. While the concept that I could somehow be responsible for other people's deaths at the hospital will seem grandiose to some, the feeling of infectiousness which I carried with me after being told I was HIV-positive in the early 1980s had certainly affected my confidence, on a range of levels, most particularly in my sexual relations with other gay men. It was common through that period for many gay men not to get tested for their HIV status because of concerns about confidentiality of records, because they didn't feel they could cope with the news or because there were no treatments available at the time anyway. This meant that the few of us who did get tested as soon as the technology became available in 1984, felt a greater sense of responsibility for ensuring that we did not infect others; for some (and this must have included me, at least on a subconscious level) there was almost a feeling of being the leper, the unclean one whom others had to protect themselves from.

To help me cope with these negative feelings I became part of a support group set up in 1986 called Melbourne Positive Friends. It was a group of HIV-positive guys who wanted to talk about the experience of being positive and the tensions it had introduced into our lives. At that stage most of us were reasonably well and we used our regular weekly meeting in each other's homes to debrief about our experiences with others, particularly partners, workmates or family members when they found out about our status and to reassure ourselves that everything would be all right: somehow the right drugs would come along or we would be amongst the lucky ones that scientists were suggesting might have stronger genes to protect them from getting AIDS.

While members were beginning to get ill by the late 1980 and there had been a number of deaths by that time, the support group did not prepare me all that well for the reality of AIDS when it was upon me. When we discussed the condition early in the piece I remember people agreeing that we could not have people in the group who had developed AIDS: they would have to go somewhere else once they'd got the 'big one'. We were a group for healthy positive guys! AIDS was the big bad bogeyman to which society responded with its Grim Reaper TV advertisements and its sensationalist media coverage of the topic throughout the 1980s — even some of the people with the virus were scared away from fully understanding what it was like to have the condition!

To be told you had AIDS was scary and, at first, for me, lonely. I knew the figures: the average lifespan for people from their first AIDS-defining illness at that time (1989) was eleven months. The doctors agreed that I might have three years of reasonable quality health if I was lucky. I was to expect to get an array of other AIDS conditions given that my T-cells had now plummeted to only ten and, while the drug AZT had been introduced and often gave some hope of extending life, it was not a cure.

So, left in my little hospital bed to contemplate my lot for the next two, maybe three years, I think it is understandable why my mind went into panic mode. I was also traumatised at the thought of rejection by my family both for being gay and now having AIDS. I was sorry that I had not had the courage to prepare my family for the possibility that I might get sick. My visits to my family, living in a northern Victorian country town, had often been only relatively quick visits over Easter or Christmas and they had not been conducive to heavy personal pronouncements. While I got on well with all of my siblings, I was nervous about the possible reactions of my conservative brothers-in-law. I had endured one too many poofter jokes over the Christmas dinner table and I was worried about the repercussions if they were to find out my secrets.

After I made that phone call from Fairfield Hospital to tell my mother I was gay and was in hospital with AIDS, I gather the family did go into a form of shock. They were unclear what to do: should they come and visit me, would they be welcome in this foreign environment? While my eldest brother who lived in Melbourne was visiting me regularly (a point which didn't seem to register amidst my mental turmoil) and my family had spoken with me over the phone on a number of occasions, I was frightened that their lack of presence at my bedside was a sign that they were rejecting me. Hence the elaborate mental story I had constructed about how the hospital was not allowing my family to visit me. They wanted to but they were stopped by the police and others at the barricades!

Several weeks later my mother and my two sisters came down to see me when I was discharged from hospital and we cleared up some of the misconceptions I'd developed during my hospital stay. They had been ringing the hospital every day and been told that I was perfectly fine: I certainly was not dying and was recovering very well from the PCP. I had not always had these phone messages passed on to me by hospital staff so I interpreted the irregular with my family as a sign that something was amiss.

That particular meeting was to herald a real change in my relations with my family. As so often happens when families undergo some sort of health crisis for one of their members, we became a lot closer and more honest about our feelings. My sister admitted that it was difficult learning that her brother had AIDS and she was conscious that the gossips in the country town where they live might spread the news in a vicious way. But she had told her husband and he was fine about it: he was just concerned that I got back on my feet again as soon as possible. It was the same with the rest of my family. I wrote a long letter to my father apologising for not preparing him better for this news and saying that I hoped he could accept that I had done nothing to hurt him or discredit the family.

My mother was soon to become part of a support group for parents of positive people, organised by Melbourne woman Joan Golding. The group met on a regular basis at the local church hall. Mum was to meet a surprising number of parents from the district who had either lost a son or daughter to AIDS or who were helping to care for them through the illness. This experience also helped her a lot to reconcile ambivalent feelings she had about the 'cause' of my sexuality: like many mothers whose children come out to them as gay, she had wondered what role she had had to play in it, had she done something wrong? She learnt to be quite comfortable with the subject with me and became close to a number of my gay friends as a result.

The support I was to receive from my friends and family in the months after my diagnosis was incredibly important in helping me to regain my strength and adopt a more positive approach to living with the condition. I even decided to go back to my work as a publications editor. My boss was a gay man too and my work colleagues had proven themselves early in the piece to be supportive around HIV. While I was nervous for a little while in the mid 1980s when jokes about coffee cups and mosquitoes spreading AIDS had been dropped occasionally, I decided to take the personal risk and tell each of my workmates, one by one, about my positive diagnosis. As a middle-level manager I needed to have the confidence of my staff and to clear up any issues they might have had. I received total support and I found that, even with some of the more socially conservative staff members, when I discussed the facts about AIDS upfront there was no difficulty; rather, a concern for my wellbeing.

I continued at work for the best part of a year but was finding my energy levels flagging to such an extent that I was rushing up to the sick bay to catch quick naps during my lunch break and was constantly finding myself nodding off during some of the important management meetings I was participating in. And anyway, I told myself, if I did only have a short time left to live as my doctors were telling me, what was I doing cooped up inside an office when I should getting out there travelling, seeing the world and enjoying myself — while I still could? I was fortunate to be a part of a good superannuation scheme with the Victorian Superannuation Board and, with a diagnosis of AIDS on my medical records, was placed on an ill-health retirement pension with a flick of the medical officer's pen.

I knew from other friends who had retired from work that the process of moving from an eight-hour structured day of activity to completely free time needed some thought and planning. While it was easy to think about filling in my time travelling overseas, going to the movies and catching up on reading, that was not necessarily going to fill in the rest of my life. I had seen friends retire from work and spend their days listlessly waiting for something to happen to their health and, in many cases, it often did. One perceptive friend described it as the 'pointing the bone' syndrome: you were told you were going to get sick and die and without some of the purpose and even the social support which work or a career provided, your illness became the central focus of your life, with death seemingly the inevitable outcome.

Not that I'm suggesting that most people with AIDS I have known died because they didn't have enough activity to fill up their lives or that they succumbed to the illness because they didn't have the right attitude.

We're talking about an incurable killer virus here which has killed some of the strongest and cleverest people I have known with no particular predicting factors about who would get sick early or who might survive for longer.

For some reason I have been one of the lucky ones who have survived much longer than the predictions. While there are still a large number of people with HIV who have still not developed AIDS even after (in some cases) fifteen years of infection, there are only a handful of people like myself who have lived for close to nine years with Category 4 AIDS. I don't pretend to know why this has been the case. Some people will say that I have had a positive attitude and that I am rarely gloomy about my prospects. To this I can say that I have been blessed with the ability to deny the statistics or the predictions any real place in my life. I don't actually believe I'm about to die and, except for the temporary psychotic episode, have not thought I was even close to meeting my Maker. A bit of healthy denial probably has helped a lot of people with supposedly terminal illnesses live quite a bit longer.

I have led a full and interesting life since leaving my job, due partly to my involvement with the Victorian AIDS Council and as a spokesperson for People Living with HIV/AIDS Victoria. In a time when it was difficult to find someone prepared to identify as a person with AIDS before the glare of the media cameras, I ignored the real risks of discrimination and bigotry and spoke to the newspapers and television about the experience of living with the virus. Surprisingly I cannot recount any stories of anything adverse happening to me because of this publicity. The worst thing that I can think of was hearing that my father had been contacted by a naturopath after an interview with me appeared in his local paper. This character claimed to Dad to have the remedy that would help me overcome my affliction! My father laughed it off, having learnt, like the rest of my family, to not be overly concerned about what people might think about my having AIDS.

I have had a series of further AIDS illnesses which have involved hospitalisation and regular visits to the outpatients department. These illnesses have included Mycobacterium Avium Complex (MAC), a relation to the bacterium that causes tuberculosis and cryptosporidiosis, caused by an intestinal parasite quite commonly found in water supplies and the pathogen behind occasional bouts of diarrhoea bugs in the community. People with normal immune systems come into contact with these bugs on a daily basis with no serious effect but for AIDS patients these can have severe and life-threatening implications. I count myself lucky though to have had a disease repertoire limited to these few conditions, even if they had downright unpleasant symptoms at the time. I say this because I have responded well to treatments for these particular conditions and only have had to add a few extra prophylactic pills to my daily intake. (I'm up to 35 tablets at present and occasionally I feel like I rattle when I walk!) I have been spared, thus far anyway, some of the very medically-dependent AIDS conditions which have really tested the patience of friends of mine; conditions like cytomegalovirus retinitis which can cause blindness and which involves infusions of fairly toxic drugs three times a week, or Kaposi's Sarcoma, the rare and sometimes unsightly cancer which can require massive doses of chemotherapy or radiotherapy to try to control its progress. I am grateful that I haven't had to attend hospital outpatients so often that it feels like a second home. Such a regular focus on your medical requirements cannot help but become tiresome for people — although I know some individuals who so enjoy the supportive atmosphere and the warm strokes they receive from nurses at Melbourne's Alfred Hospital that they actually look forward to their regular visits. For my lot I could do without such intrusions into my busy timetable!

The most important reason why I am still here to tell my story though is undoubtedly the advances in HIV/AIDS treatments which have continued through much of the 1990s. While they were too late for many of my friends and still do not work for a significant percentage of people, the triple antiviral therapy, which has become the gold standard for HIV/AIDS treatments at the moment, is transforming the health of so many of my friends that to describe it as 'miraculous' and 'amazing' does not seem far short of the mark. People with advanced disease have often been able to halt further deterioration and see their T-cell counts rise and viral load counts plummet. (Viral load tests are a recently introduced technology which measure the amount of HIV that is active in the blood.) Individuals who, on medical predictions before the therapies would not have survived for longer than a year or so, have turned around their health outlooks, added weight and strength and, in some cases, have gone back to work.

While we have all been told that the prospect of resistance developing to the therapies after a few years is very real, people now have hope that they will remain well long enough to be around for the next drug or medical advance. Hope is in the air, albeit tinged with enough uncertainty to make one careful not to say that the AIDS crisis is over; the dramas and difficulties which this virus has brought into some people's lives have not gone away.

As I write this I have learnt of the death of a good friend of mine after a valiant battle for the past year or so with a voracious AIDS illness. Tomorrow I will attend his funeral and, while it is hard to admit this, the grief and loss I feel at his passing will be somewhat numbed by the experience of the past few years. People in the HIV community have lost so many friends and become so accustomed to attending funerals and memorial services that the hurt has often been pushed somewhere into our subconscious. Some people have said that, if there is ever a definite cure found for this virus, that is when people's walls of defence will come tumbling down, that they will be able to put the grief of this epidemic into some sort of perspective and the real tears will flow. I can hardly wait for the day — but I'm going to try!

Index